Treat Your Own Knees

"[This book] provides a safe and effective plan for improving range of motion and strength for anyone with either an acute or a chronic knee-joint problem."

— James R. Roberson, M.D.
Professor and chairman, Department of Orthopaedics
Emory University Medical School

Treat Your Own Knees

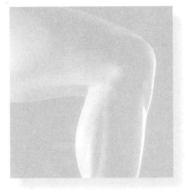

Jim Johnson, P.T.

Hunter House
PUBLISHERS

Hunter House Inc., Publishers
PO Box 2914
Alameda CA 94501-0914

Library of Congress Cataloging-in-Publication Data
Johnson, Jim, P.T.
Treat your own knees / Jim Johnson.
p. cm.
Includes bibliographical references and index.
ISBN-13: 978-0-89793-422-0 (pbk.) – ISBN-10: 0-89793-422-9 (pbk.)
1. Knee—Care and hygiene. 2. Knee—Wounds and injuries. I. Title.
RD561.J6285 2003
617.5′82—dc21   2003012853

Project Credits
Cover Design: Peri Poloni, Knockout Books
Book Production: Jinni Fontana Graphic Design
Exercise Illustrator: Eunice Johnson
Copy Editor: Kelley Blewster
Proofreader: John David Marion
Indexer: Nancy D. Peterson
Acquisitions Editor: Jeanne Brondino
Editor: Alexandra Mummery
Publicist: Lisa E. Lee
Foreign Rights Assistant: Elisabeth Wohofsky
Customer Service Manager: Christina Sverdrup
Order Fulfillment: Lakdhon Lama
Administrator: Theresa Nelson
Computer Support: Peter Eichelberger
Publisher: Kiran S. Rana

Printed and Bound by Bang Printing, Brainerd, Minnesota
Manufactured in the United States of America

9 8 7   First Edition   08 09 10 11 12

Contents

Foreword

The knee is a complex structure subjected to heavy repetitive loads. It is no surprise that the joint is frequently injured, prompting the need for expert advice on how to rehabilitate it.

Jim Johnson's book is a clearly written, easy-to-understand guide for the person without a medical background. It provides a safe and effective plan for improving range of motion and strength for anyone with either an acute or a chronic knee-joint problem. Those dealing with a less-than-perfect knee joint will find this information to be educational and helpful.

— James R. Roberson, M.D.
Professor and chairman, Department of Orthopaedics
Emory University Medical School

Please note: I have given my best effort to ensure that this book is entirely based upon scientific evidence and *not* on intuition, single case reports, opinions of authorities, anecdotal evidence, or unsystematic clinical observations. Where I do offer my opinion in the book, it is directly stated as such.

— Jim Johnson, P.T.

Acknowledgments

I have always thought that the making of a book is quite similar to the building of a house. It is not there because one man built it all by himself; rather it is the result of a group of individuals working together. As the author, I see myself as the "architect" who drew up the plans.

In and of themselves, however, plans are worthless unless put into action by a skillful construction team, which, in this case, is the staff at Hunter House. I would like to thank each and every person who was involved one way or another, be it big or small, in the production of this book. It simply would not have been possible without them. Also, a special thanks to James Griffing at ExRx.com for his assistance in locating some of the pictures used in the book.

And last, but certainly not least, I owe a big "thank you" to my wife, Cathy. Let it be known that I only had the luxury of writing this book because she was busy "holding the front lines" by doing less exciting things such as the laundry and helping the kids with their homework. She is in essence "the glue" holding the family together, and for that I am extremely lucky and thankful.

Important Note

The material in this book is intended to provide a review of information regarding the treatment of knee pain. Every effort has been made to provide accurate and dependable information. The contents of this book have been compiled through professional research and in consultation with medical professionals. However, health-care professionals have differing opinions, and advances in medical and scientific research are made very quickly, so some of the information may become outdated.

Therefore, the publisher, author, and editors and the professionals quoted in the book cannot be held responsible for any error, omission, or dated material. The author and publisher assume no responsibility for any outcome of applying the information in this book in a program of self-care or under the care of a licensed practitioner. If you have questions concerning your knees, or about the application of the information described in this book, consult a qualified health-care professional.

Introduction

My name is Jim and I'm a physical therapist. I work full-time in a large teaching hospital where most of the day I can be found wrangling with patients' aches and pains. Many problems I can solve, but in all honesty some leave me scratching my head. One may wonder why a person who makes his living from treating patients would want to write a book showing people how to treat their own knee problems. It's a fair question, and I'll do my best to answer it.

There are two good reasons why I wrote this book. The first is a matter of people's time and convenience. Many people are busy working full-time or raising a family (or both), and while physical therapy is very important, it simply may not be feasible for these individuals. I have seen many, many patients over the years who could have definitely benefited from supervised physical therapy but who could only come to see me one time to get some advice and learn some exercises because that was the best their busy schedules afforded.

The second reason is cost. For a lot of people, paying regular visits to a physical therapist means missing time from work. Then there can be child-care concerns, transportation to physical therapy, and perhaps parking fees. Sometimes other direct costs, such as insurance copayments or perhaps buying therapy equipment such as ankle weights or ice packs that may or may not be covered by insurance, may enter the picture.

Now don't get me wrong. There are indeed lots of knee problems that absolutely need direct care by a physical therapist, and patients must make it a priority to get to their appointments in those cases. However, after more than a decade of treating hundreds of patients, I have come to realize that a good many people have simple, straightforward knee problems and that all they really need is a good home-exercise program. Following a program like the one suggested in *Treat Your Own Knees* would have saved these individuals much time and money.

This brings us to the next issue: exactly whom this book is written for. Of course it's written for persons with knee pain, but I can tell you from clinical experience that not all knee pain is the same. Serious knee problems, while uncommon, exist and must be dealt with. Writing this book, I am at a disadvantage in that I do not know every reader's medical history. This is where your doctor comes in. I recommend that every reader see a physician to get medical clearance to follow the program outlined in this book. Then, after a doctor's okay, dive right in.

In my opinion, the following is a list of individuals who will likely benefit *the most* from this book:

◆ those suffering knee pain that appeared without any known cause and has been plaguing them for a while;

◆ people with knee arthritis;

◆ people with persistent knee pain who have tried just about everything under the sun to get rid of it, to no avail;

◆ people who experience knee pain despite having a normal-appearing X ray and physical examination by a doctor.

While this book is written for the average person with knee pain whose treatment involves no special equipment, the exact same treatment principles would be used to treat athletes. The only thing that might change would be the use of either more sophisticated equipment or higher-level exercises. To that end, I have included some exercise substitutions in Chapter 7.

Don't worry if you don't find yourself fitting exactly into any of the above categories. It's just a list of who might potentially get the most from the information in this book. The real beauty of this program is that it treats the function of the knee, rather than treating any given diagnosis. Therefore, as long as your doctor has given you the go-ahead, I am not necessarily concerned with whether you have arthritis, a torn meniscus, or whatever, but rather with other things, such as how well your knee bends or how strong certain knee-related muscles are. Due to the fact that the true source of knee pain is unknown in a fair number of cases, and that a significant percentage of people are walking around with structural abnormalities in their knee yet don't experience knee pain, I have found this approach to be a very practical and useful way to attack knee problems.

Some readers may be skeptically asking at this point, "But can a home program really work?" You bet it can. And let me tell you this. When I say something works, I don't say it based upon my personal experience or anecdotal evidence. I will only say a treatment works when it has been proven effective in a controlled trial, or better yet in a randomized controlled trial (more on those later). As a for-instance, take the randomized controlled trial that was published in the October 2002 issue of the renowned *British Medical Journal*. It involved 786 men and women with knee pain who participated in a simple home-based exercise program (quite similar to the one in this book) designed to improve strength, range of motion, and function. The study demonstrated without question that the program was quite capable of significantly reducing knee pain.

Yet other people may have thumbed through this book and be quite surprised at how simple the exercises are, such as the knee-strengthening exercise that uses nothing more sophisticated than a common pillow. They may wonder, "How could such a simple little exercise really help that much?" Please be assured that each exercise in this book was specifically included on the basis of its simplicity, its practicality, the ease with which it can be performed, and how much research was available to back up its use. As an example, when I considered all factors, it was a well-done clinical trial that swayed me to use an isometric strengthening exercise (i.e., an exercise involving pushing into an immovable object, such as a wall) as opposed to a more dynamic one (such as the use of a leg-press machine) to strengthen the knee. Published in the peer-reviewed journal *The Archives of Physical Medicine and Rehabilitation* was a randomized controlled trial that compared the effectiveness of isometric exercise to that of the more popularly used dynamic type, which in this case involved the use of elastic bands for resistance. One hundred two patients with knee arthritis participated in this study, which proved that the seemingly puny isometric mode of exercise could strengthen the knee of the knee-pain patient every bit as much as the more dynamic kind of exercise, without all the fuss of using more complicated exercise equipment.

But enough about controlled trials for now. More examples concerning these trials will pop up throughout the book, so you can have every confidence that what I say is firmly rooted in the latest scientific research. Again, I have given my best effort to ensuring that the book is based entirely on scientific evidence rather than on intuition, single case reports, opinions of authorities, anecdotal evidence, or unsystematic clinical observations. Where I do offer my opinion in the book, it is directly stated as such.

This is an action book, and now is the time to get started. I've sifted through piles of knee research, field-tested the exercises, and done all the groundwork to bring you this simple program, which you can carry out at home without special equipment. All you have to do is keep the pages turning and put forth your best effort. As the great Will Rogers once said, "Even if you're on the right track, you'll get run over if you just sit there."

1

The Four Abilities Your Knee Must Have

Each time someone with knee pain comes to see me, I keep one thought in the back of my mind: The pain is most likely the result of something that is functioning improperly. My job as a physical therapist is not necessarily to come up with the exact cause of someone's pain (which can often be either elusive or controversial), but rather to figure out what the knee isn't doing that it normally should do. Using this approach during my evaluation, I test the various knee functions—such as how strong the muscles are or how far the patient can bend the knee—so I can determine what is or is not working up to par. Once the improper function has been identified, I can then choose a treatment that will restore it.

Consider the following list of the possible treatments for knee pain:

- hot packs
- arthroscopy
- manual therapy
- total knee replacement
- range-of-motion exercises

- proprioception exercises
- strengthening exercises
- electrical stimulation
- ultrasound
- ice packs
- whirlpool
- exercise bike/treadmill/walking
- massage
- mind-body techniques
- joint aspiration/injections
- pain medicines

As you can see from this rather lengthy list, medicine has developed quite a wide range of treatment options when it comes to solving the problem of knee pain, and I am sure that many more will evolve as time passes. Although some of them appear to be markedly different from others, they all have a common thread running through them: *Each of them is designed to restore or enhance the functioning of the knee area.*

Take a moment to think about this. Ice reduces the swelling in your knee so you can bend it easier (and in turn, it hurts a lot less). Strengthening exercises provide stability to the knee by making the muscles stronger. Walking improves the ability of the muscles to move the knee repeatedly. The most radical treatment, total knee replacement, improves the function of the entire knee area by putting in a new joint that can bend and straighten with ease.

Thinking in this manner about treatments for knee pain can be quite useful when one is trying to figure out which is the best treatment method to use. As an example, if a knee is unable to bend as far as it should, a treatment is needed that will improve the knee's range of motion. And if one of the leg muscles is found to be weak, then a strengthening exercise would be in order. These, then, are the underlying principles upon which this book is based.

Most knee pain is the result of dysfunction. Restore the function with the proper treatment and your pain will be relieved.

Proper Knee Function: The Four Abilities of Your Knee

Although your knee may seem like a simple hinge joint that swings back and forth as you go about your daily routine, it is really one of your body's more complex joints. If you were able to look beneath the skin and underlying fat near the knee, the first thing you would lay your eyes on would be the muscles around the knee. Figures 1.1 and 1.2 (on the facing page) are drawings of the major muscles in the upper leg. These are the muscles that primarily affect knee movement.

As you can see from these diagrams, many different muscles surround your knee. Think of these muscles as the "engines" that make it possible for you to move your legs. For instance, when you want to stand up, your leg muscles respond by quickly contracting and getting shorter. As this happens, they pull on the bones they are attached to, thus enabling you to move to a standing position. This brings us to the first ability your knee must have: *strength*. A knee with good muscular strength can adequately perform what it is being called upon to do (such as climbing stairs), while keeping the joint in a safe and stable position.

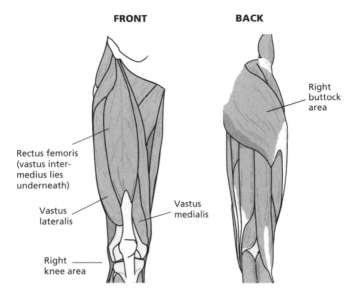

FRONT   BACK

Right buttock area

Rectus femoris (vastus intermedius lies underneath)

Vastus lateralis

Vastus medialis

Right knee area

Figures 1.1 and 1.2 The major muscles of the upper leg and the knee area

Let's say we continued with our anatomical investigation and removed all of the leg muscles. What would we be looking at then? We would be looking at the bones and the actual knee joint itself. Figure 1.3 (on the next page) is a close-up view of the knee joint and all of its major ligaments:

Looks a little more complicated than just a plain old hinge, doesn't it? While the knee joint itself is made up of some sophisticated-looking structures, it really has one simple job: to allow movement freely in several directions. This motion, although smaller in range than that of the hip or shoulder joint, is essential in order to accomplish many of the things we do each day. When I worked full-time on an orthopedic floor in a large teaching hospital, I occasionally treated patients who had their knee joint surgically fused due to trauma or an infection. It was then that I began to appreciate just how important the motion at the knee really is and how much we take it for granted. For these patients, performing even the simplest of tasks that most people effortlessly do each day, such as walking or rising from a chair, became very cumbersome due to this lost motion. The next time you get out of bed in the morning, try doing it with your knee perfectly straight and you'll see what I mean. This makes *flexibility* the second requirement for a healthy, functioning knee.

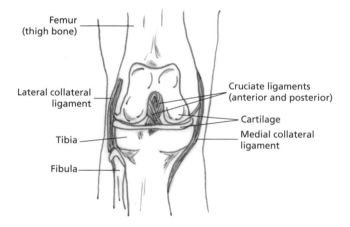

Femur
(thigh bone)

Lateral collateral
ligament

Tibia

Fibula

Cruciate ligaments
(anterior and posterior)

Cartilage

Medial collateral
ligament

Figure 1.3 Right knee joint

Too detailed to include in the above illustrations are all the tiny nerves that go to the knee area. Without giving you an anatomy lesson, let me say that the nerves in your body are divided into two kinds: sensory nerves and motor nerves. Motor nerves travel from your brain down to your knee (as well as to other areas of the body) and allow you to control the muscles so you can move your knee (or other body parts). Sensory nerves, on the other hand, go in exactly the opposite direction from the motor nerves. They travel from your knee (or other areas of the body) back up to your brain. Since their job is to carry and report sensations—such as hot or cold—they must travel to your brain so you can be constantly aware of what is going on in your knee (or elsewhere). Some of the most important information that these sensory nerves carry are messages regarding the position your knee is in. Small nerves in your knee's muscles, tendons, and joint capsule (the covering around the knee joint) all provide information to your brain as to the position and movement of your knee. This is known as *proprioception*.

To get a better idea of what proprioception is and its purpose, try this simple test: Sit or lie perfectly still. Close your eyes. Can you tell if your knee is bent or straight? If your legs are crossed, is the right over the left, or is the left over the right? Like most people, you probably have a good idea of what position your legs are in and how bent or straight they are—even with your eyes closed. This is a good example of proprioception in action, and it is made possible by the sensory nerves in your knee. Because they send precise information to your brain about your knee's position, you are able to correctly determine its position. Since every knee needs this ability to properly function, *proprioception* takes an important spot at number three on our list of requirements for a healthy knee.

Completing the list is *endurance*. Endurance is the ability of your knee to do its job not just one or two times, but over and over and over again. Examples are numerous and include activities such as walking, running, and stair climbing. While we are doing these kinds of tasks, we ask our knees to bend and straighten many times in a row. If our knees fail to keep up with the job, several things can happen. The muscles will start to tire and might become unable to keep the knee joint within a safe range of stability while it is moving. The knee can then start to buckle (or snap back too far, for that matter) and stress the delicate structures. Given either enough time or a poorly conditioned knee, the muscles can grow fatigued and simply give up. It is at this point that you will be unable to walk the whole distance you want to or make it to the top of the stairs. Thus, endurance is a must-have for full knee functioning and becomes the fourth ability your knee must have.

> **The Four Abilities Your Knee Must Have**
> - *good muscular strength*
> - *adequate flexibility*
> - *working proprioception*
> - *enough endurance to allow it to perform movements over and over again*

The Game Plan

As stated in the beginning of this chapter, most knee pain is the result of a loss of function. That is, something in your knee is not working as it should. Therefore, if we restore the function, the pain will subside. This is where the four abilities your knee must have fit into the picture. Chapters 2 through 5 are each devoted to one of the abilities of a healthy knee. By doing the specific exercises included in those chapters, you will be able to restore any of the four abilities that your knee has lost, directly improving the functioning of your knee. Doing so in turn will equal relief from pain. Chapter 6, titled "Some Things You May *Not* Have Thought About," addresses a few additional issues regarding knee health and knee pain, and offers a mind-body technique proven to help ease pain. Chapter 7 pulls everything together into an easy-to-follow weekly program.

The following is a diagram that represents the overall approach you will be using when treating your own knee:

The Game Plan

Normally functioning, pain-free knee

Good strength
Adequate flexibility
Intact proprioception
Ample endurance

↓

**Trauma, accidents,
and aging changes**

↓

Loss of function

*Knee loses one or more of the four abilities:
strength, proprioception, flexibility, or endurance*

↓

Pain

↓

*Regain function by doing specific exercises to
restore the four abilities*

↓

Pain-free again

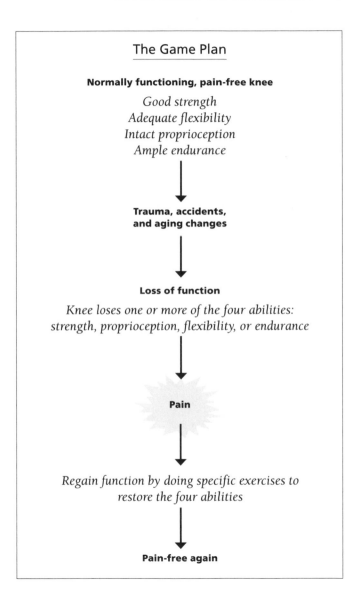

2

If You Strengthen Just One Knee Muscle, Make Sure It's This One

It would be quite hard for you to do much at all without the help of your muscles. Even something as basic and simple as walking requires the forces from no fewer than twenty-eight of your leg muscles in order for you to carefully control the pull of gravity as you try to move forward. As stated earlier, muscles act as "engines" that your body uses to make itself move. The following is a list of some of the muscles that are situated in and around the knee area:

- ◆ sartorius
- ◆ gracilis
- ◆ adductor magnus and longus
- ◆ the quadriceps—vastus lateralis, medialis, intermedius, and rectus femoris
- ◆ the hamstrings—semimembranosus, semitendinosus, and biceps femoris
- ◆ gastrocnemius
- ◆ popliteus

You can see that there are many leg muscles with unusual names. They all play a part one way or another in the functioning of our knees. However, many studies over the years have pointed out that some of these muscles clearly deserve more attention than others when it comes to knee problems. It appears as though some muscles, for various reasons, are "hit harder" when you have a problem with your knee. Strangely enough, some muscles are able to continue working adequately in the face of swelling or sudden injury to the knee, while others respond by getting weaker or smaller, or by shutting down altogether. For the purposes of this book, you can take this as really good news. It means that you will not have to spend a lot of time doing countless exercises to strengthen each of the individual muscles in the knee area.

A Selective Problem

Over the years, I have spent a great deal of time in the medical library, trying to find out exactly what knee conditions affect which muscles. When I initially started my investigation in this area, I expected the research to show, for example, that arthritis caused problems mainly for one or two muscles, while a torn ligament took its toll on a completely different muscle. What I found, however, was rather surprising. It quickly became apparent that for just about every single knee condition I was checking out (such as arthritis, ligament tears, etc.) *the same muscle* kept cropping up over and over as being the one most affected. And just what muscle was it?

In the cadaver lab back in physical therapy school we learned the muscle's Latin name, *musculus quadriceps femoris*. Most doctors and physical therapists, however, commonly call it the *quadriceps*, which literally translates into "four-headed muscle." If you're like me and prefer nicknames, you can just call it "the quads."

The quads are indeed made up of four distinct muscles. They are the following:

- ◆ vastus lateralis
- ◆ vastus medialis
- ◆ vastus intermedius
- ◆ rectus femoris

The first three muscles, vastus lateralis, vastus medialis, and vastus intermedius, all attach themselves to the bone of your upper leg, cross your knee in the front, and then attach to the big bone in your lower leg. The last one, rectus femoris, attaches itself a little bit differently. It starts your hip area, just below your belt line in the front, and then continues down to cross your knee like the other three vastus muscles.

Figure 2.1 is a close-up illustration of the quads, looking at the right leg from the front. Note that you can only see three of the four muscles of the quadriceps, as the vastus intermedius lies neatly buried under the rectus femoris.

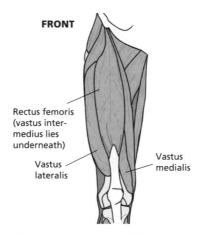

FRONT

Rectus femoris (vastus intermedius lies underneath)

Vastus lateralis

Vastus medialis

Figure 2.1 The Quadriceps (Quads) Muscle Group

So just what do the quads do? Well, if you're sitting in a chair at the moment, kick out your leg. This action is one of the main jobs of the quads; that is, they help you straighten out your leg. Now try this. Stand up from a sitting position, and as you do so, put one hand onto the front of your thigh. You should be able to feel the muscles under your hand (the quads) tighten and firm up as you begin to rise. This is yet another important function of this muscle. With your foot fixed on the floor as you stand up, the quads work to pull you into a standing position. Along with these activities, your quads are also largely responsible for your ability to walk, run, jump, and climb stairs. Additionally, the knee joint itself depends heavily on the quads to help stabilize and support it.

> *Knee problems tend to cause isolated muscle wasting and weakness, specifically in the quadriceps group.*

Effects of Various Knee Problems on the Quads

Let's take a brief look at the evidence from peer-reviewed journals that have shown the quadriceps to be selectively affected by a variety of knee conditions. (Peer-reviewed journals are magazines that only publish articles that have been reviewed by experts in the field.) The chances are good that most readers will fit into one of the following categories.

◆ ◆ ◆ *Knee Swelling and the Quadriceps*

Experiencing swelling in your knee has been shown to be a major reason why your quads might not be working like they should. If you were to lie flat on your back as I injected a harmless salt-water solution known as *saline* into your knee, you would find that after a certain amount of this fluid entered your knee joint, you would no longer be able to lift your leg off the table. Then, as I removed the saline a little at a time, you would slowly start to regain control of your leg once again and be able to lift it. Here's what some of the studies that have looked into this unusual effect of having extra fluid in the knee joint have found:

◆ One study took patients with chronic (long-term) knee swelling, removed the excess fluid using a needle, and measured an immediate increase in quadriceps strength (Fahrer 1988).

◆ Another study demonstrated that even if you have as little as 20 milliliters of fluid in your knee (which is just over a tablespoon), it's enough to decrease the strength of your quadriceps muscle (Spencer 1984).

As you can see, it takes a whole lot less than a huge, swollen knee in order to prevent your quadriceps muscle from working properly. According to the research, having just over a tablespoon of fluid in the knee—probably too small an amount for most people to visibly notice—is sufficient to trigger a problem.

◆ ◆ ◆ *Knee Injuries and the Quadriceps*

Several studies have taken a close look at how the muscles of the leg respond to a knee injury. Two physical therapists from the University of Delaware, Tara Manal and Lynn Snyder-Mackler, specifically examined people who had recently fallen on their knee or sustained a direct blow to their kneecap (such as being hit with a hockey stick or striking the knee on the dashboard during a car accident). Their results showed that only about two-thirds of these individuals had a properly contracting quadriceps muscle following the injury.

Along the same lines, but in a more sophisticated study (Young 1980), the quadriceps muscle of people with a history of knee injury was examined in greater detail. By using an ultrasound machine, pictures could be taken of the individual leg muscles and the size of each one could be assessed. Subjects in the study had a wide range of diagnoses, including

- ♦ surgical removal of part of the knee cartilage
- ♦ various knee injuries
- ♦ fractured tibia (a lower leg bone)
- ♦ surgical opening of the knee joint
- ♦ pes anserinus (tendon) transfer

Additionally, each subject had their mid-thigh circumference measured with a tape measure to detect any differences between legs. As one would expect, in most cases, the injured leg was smaller around than the noninjured leg, possibly indicating that some of the muscles had wasted away due to the injury. The exact muscles involved, however, could not be determined with a simple tape-measurement technique. It took the aid of the ultrasound pictures for the researchers to accurately tell that the muscle-wasting process was largely due to just one muscle—the quadriceps.

♦ ♦ ♦ *Ligament Problems and the Quadriceps*

Ligaments are tough fibrous tissues that attach bones to each other. One of their primary functions is to stabilize joints. Problems with the ligaments in the knee can spell trouble for the quadriceps muscle. In particular, the *anterior cruciate ligament* and the *medial collateral ligament* have been the subject of much research. (See Figure 1.2 for detailed pictures of these ligaments.)

Known most popularly as the *ACL*, the anterior cruciate ligament controls motion between the lower leg bone, the tibia, and the upper leg bone, the femur. A lot of anterior cruciate injuries occur when the knee is forcefully twisted or hyperextended (bent backwards), which can tear and even rupture this ligament. If the rip is severe enough, the knee joint can eventually become unstable, leading to what most orthopedic surgeons refer to as "an instability."

A 1985 study in *The Journal of Bone and Joint Surgery* took a group of forty-one patients headed to surgery due to an instability of the anterior cruciate ligament and examined their knee muscles through images obtained by CT scans. CT, or computed tomography, scans use computers to create special three-dimensional pictures from flat X rays. In this way, the researchers could directly assess what toll the instability of the anterior cruciate ligament had taken on the knee muscles. It was found that of all the thigh muscles, the quadriceps wasted away the most by far.

The study did not follow these patients to see how the quadriceps muscle fared after surgery to repair the injured ligament, but others have. In one study (Lopresti 1984), thirteen athletes were followed for a full year after undergoing surgical repair of the anterior cruciate ligament. Once again, CT scans of both legs were taken. True to form, the quadriceps showed selective wasting away compared to the other muscles, with a noted 15 percent reduction from its normal size.

In addition to the anterior cruciate ligament, the medial collateral ligament has also been investigated. This ligament is located along the inner part of the knee and sits vertically across the joint rather like a piece of tape holding the two leg bones together. Its job is to prevent the knee from buckling inward; it is commonly injured when a force is applied to the outside of the knee, as in a football clipping injury.

A clever study from Sweden done in the early sixties (Stener 1962) took thirty subjects with partial ruptures of the medial collateral ligament and carefully examined them with an electromyography (EMG) machine, which picks up the electrical activity of muscles. By hooking up some of the muscles around the knee to the EMG machine and then recording their electrical activity as tension was applied to the ruptured ligament (ouch!), the researchers could tell exactly how the muscles reacted when the medial collateral ligament was torn.

These researchers found that of all the muscles tested, it was only the vastus medialis (which is part of the quadriceps muscle group) that showed no electrical response while the researchers were stretching this ligament. It would appear, then, that for all practical purposes, the quadriceps can have a tendency to "shut down" with this type of knee injury.

◆ ◆ ◆ *Knee Pain and the Quadriceps*

Bertil Stener (1969), of the University of Goteborg in Sweden, reported an interesting case study that illustrates just how effectively pain can cause a major loss of quadriceps strength.

A forty-five-year-old man went to the doctor one day complaining of a three-year history of pain in his right knee. Upon examining the knee, the doctor found that the patient had a firm lump, about half the size of a walnut, on the outer part of his knee, as well as severe wasting away of the entire quadriceps muscle group. X-ray tests were ordered, which subsequently revealed the lump to be a tumor.

The most interesting thing about this case is that although the man could move his knee forward and backward rather freely, the pain occurred only at certain angles of knee bending, mainly in the thirty- to sixty-degree range. In other words, when the knee was perfectly straight there was no pain, but as the man kept bending his knee, a terrible pain set in once he bent it in the range of thirty to sixty degrees. Oddly enough, after the knee was bent past the sixty-degree mark, the pain vanished.

Stener guessed that the pain occurred only in the thirty- to sixty-degree range because it was probably during this angle of knee bending that a structure called the *iliotibial band* (a thick band of tissue that goes across the side of the knee joint) was able to slide over the bony tumor and cause the pain. He also theorized that the wasting away of the quadriceps muscle was largely due to the frequent pain that prevented the quads from contracting properly.

To test his theory, Stener had the patient hooked up to an EMG machine as he sat on the edge of a table. With the leg hanging freely, the man was asked to straighten his leg (the main function of the quadriceps, as you will recall) and then keep it straight. Pressure was then applied to the tumor at the side of his knee. This pressure, of course, caused terrible knee pain, and as soon as the discomfort was felt, the man's quadriceps muscle suddenly gave out, rendering him totally incapable of holding his leg straight out. EMG analysis confirmed these observations and showed that two muscles of the quadriceps group, the vastus medialis and vastus lateralis, were particularly affected by the painful stimulus.

The patient eventually had the tumor surgically removed. Seven weeks after the operation, the pain disappeared and the function of the quadriceps improved rapidly, becoming a classic example of how pain in the knee can have devastating effects on certain muscles.

◆ ◆ ◆ *Knee Arthritis and the Quadriceps*

Arthritis—or more specifically *osteoarthritis*—of the knee has taken its place as one of the most common causes of chronic disability among the elderly. I have treated many patients for it and am willing to bet that many readers of this book have been diagnosed with it.

Since the condition is so widespread, you may have guessed that an enormous amount of research has been published on the topic. In order to give you all the "important stuff" without getting too bogged down in piles of research, I have chosen to summarize the information you most need to be aware of. It is as follows:

- ♦ Hassan (2001) took seventy-seven people with symptomatic knee osteoarthritis and compared them to sixty-three controls with normal knees matched for age and sex. This means that if you are a fifty-year-old woman with knee arthritis, your knees were compared to those of another fifty-year-old woman who had normal knees. Comparisons of these two groups revealed that people with knee osteoarthritis have much weaker quadriceps muscles than those with normal knees.

- ♦ Hurley (1993) looked at people who had osteoarthritis in one knee. After strength testing, it was found that the quadriceps muscle in the arthritic knee of all the subjects was consistently 30–40 percent weaker than in their normal knee.

- ♦ Studies examining the strength of the muscles around the knee in subjects with osteoarthritis repeatedly show the quadriceps to be selectively weakened (Slemenda 1997).

- ♦ Some readers may be thinking that perhaps people with knee osteoarthritis show muscle weakness in all these studies simply because it hurts when they move their knee, thus preventing them from showing their true strength. A good thought; however, when researchers study random groups of people using X rays and strength tests, quadriceps weakness also exists in persons with knee osteoarthritis who have no knee pain (Slemenda 1997).

> **The following conditions have been associated with muscle wasting and weakness in just the quadriceps:**
>
> ◆ *swelling in the knee*
> ◆ *having had surgery on the knee*
> ◆ *history of injuries, including falls or direct blows to the knee*
> ◆ *fractures of the tibia*
> ◆ *having torn knee ligaments*
> ◆ *having knee pain*
> ◆ *having arthritis in the knee*

As you can see, it is well established in the medical literature that the quadriceps muscle is clearly singled out when it comes to knee osteoarthritis. The million-dollar question, however, seems to be which comes first. Does osteoarthritis cause quadriceps weakness, or does quadriceps weakness cause osteoarthritis? Dr. Slemenda, a specialist in epidemiology at the Indiana University School of Medicine, has conducted some exciting research that may help us solve this riddle. He studied a group of 141 elderly women who were living independently and who lacked any X-ray signs of knee osteoarthritis in one or both knees. Among other variables, muscle strength of the knee muscles was assessed. Follow-up X rays were taken about two and a half years later and showed that those women who went on to develop knee osteoarthritis had 18 percent weaker quadriceps muscles *at the beginning of the study* (that is, when they showed no signs of osteoarthritis) compared to those women who continued to have normal knees. Clearly, more research is needed to draw firm conclusions, but these findings do lend strong support to the notion that quadriceps weakness comes before X-ray signs of knee osteoarthritis and is strongly predictive of someone getting it. Maybe an ounce of prevention really is worth a pound of cure!

A Surefire Way to Strengthen Your Quadriceps

Okay, enough research for now. Since we know that the majority of knee problems selectively weaken the quadriceps muscle, the next step is to get the muscle's strength back to normal. When I prescribe an exercise to accomplish this particular goal, I must take several factors into account. Above all, the exercise must have been scientifically shown in studies to (1) activate the target muscle (the quads), and (2) increase its size and strength. The next thing that needs to be addressed if I am considering a home exercise program is the patient's access to exercise equipment. Does the patient have a gym membership or any exercise machines available for his or her use? Other issues must be factored into the equation as well, such as how much range of motion is available at the knee joint. Can the patient freely move his or her knee back and forth, or is it too painful to move very much at all, making the use of most exercise machines out of the question? Indeed, all these issues and more determine which exercise I will prescribe to best meet the patient's needs.

Since this is a book, I am at a bit of a disadvantage because I haven't examined your particular knee and therefore lack the answers to the above questions. In order to get around this problem, I will give you an exercise that, although it may not be perfectly tailored for your exact knee, will most certainly make your quadriceps muscle stronger, require zero equipment, and in all likelihood agree with more then 95 percent of readers' knees.

And what exercise could possibly meet all these requirements? It's called an *isometric exercise*. The word *isometric* comes from the two Greek words *isos*, meaning "equal" or "like," and *metron*, meaning "measure." An isometric exercise, then, is one in which the length of the muscle stays the same as it is contracting. A good example of this is when you use your hand and arm to push hard against a brick wall. Your arm is still and is unable to move because you can't push the wall over, yet there is a definite building up of tension in your muscle, which can definitely make it stronger over time if the exercise is done using proper guidelines.

Don't worry, I'm not going to have you pushing on any brick walls to beef up your quadriceps muscle. Instead, we're going to use something a little gentler on the knees—a pillow. Here's what the exercise looks like:

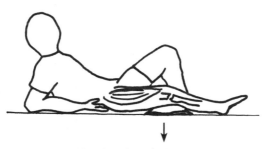

Figure 2.2 Strengthening the quadriceps

Doesn't look too hard, does it? In fact, some readers may be thinking that it looks a little too easy to do much of anything at all. Recall the first two factors that I take into account when prescribing an exercise to strengthen the quads: It must have been scientifically shown in studies to activate the target muscle and to increase its size and strength.

At least two well-done studies have proven without a doubt that this exercise is indeed a heavyweight when it comes to fighting wimpy quads. Both studies were what researchers refer to as *randomized controlled trials.* Randomized controlled trials are just what you should look for because they are considered to be the highest form of proof in medicine that a treatment is truly effective. The main reason for this is because the subjects are randomly assigned to either a treatment group (a group that does quad exercises, for example) or a control group that does nothing at all. Comparing these two groups at the end of the study allows the researchers to know for sure if the exercise (or whatever treatment is being studied) was really effective, or if the same results would have occurred anyway even without the treatment.

The first randomized controlled trial (Carolan 1992) had a group of men isometrically contract their quadriceps muscle as hard as they could, and to hold the contraction for three to four seconds. They did this exercise three days per week, thirty times per day. After eight weeks of isometric training, the subjects had increased the strength of their quadriceps by a whopping 33 percent!

The other randomized controlled trial (Garfinkel 1992) followed basically the same format, except it took things one step further. This time, females got a chance to do the exercises using essentially the same training program as in the previously mentioned study. However, these investigators not only measured strength changes in the quadriceps, they also took CT scans of the entire thigh so they could objectively determine if any muscles had actually increased in size as a result of exercising. Eight weeks later, at the conclusion of the study, subjects once again showed amazing gains in strength, with their quadriceps becoming a full 28 percent stronger. Pictures from the CT scans of the leg muscles were also highly significant, showing that the subjects' quadriceps muscles had grown 15 percent bigger.

Strengthening Your Quadriceps Muscle with Isometrics

◆ *Isometric exercise involves applying a force to an immovable object. The muscles build up tension, but there is no actual movement.*

◆ *Multiple randomized controlled trials have proven that isometrics can increase both the size and the strength of the quadriceps muscle in men and women.*

STRENGTHENING EXERCISE FOR THE QUADRICEPS MUSCLE

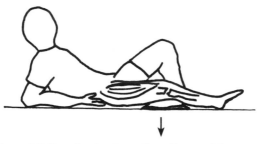

Figure 2.3 Exercise to strengthen the quadriceps

◆ Get into a position similar to the one shown in Figure 2.3. You can either recline on your elbows or lie flat on your back.

◆ Fold a pillow in half, and place it under the knee of the leg that is extended, as shown. If this doesn't feel right, you can do the exercise without the pillow and with your knee straight.

- Press down as hard as you comfortably can into the pillow with your extended knee, and hold for three to five seconds. The muscle on the top of your leg, above the kneecap (the quadriceps), should tighten up.

- Do this thirty times on the leg with the painful knee, holding each contraction for three to five seconds. Then switch and exercise the other leg if you wish. Repeat the exercise three times per week, separated by a day between sessions (either Monday-Wednesday-Friday or Tuesday-Thursday-Saturday). If necessary, work up to the thirty repetitions by adding a few more reps per session until you reach thirty.

- After eight weeks, your quads should be bigger and stronger—the research has proven it!

3

How to Restore Flexibility to Your Knee

So far we've talked about restoring the first ability every healthy knee must have: good muscular strength. While of utmost importance, strength is but one piece of the puzzle when treating knee pain. This is due to the fact that the most powerful knee muscles in the world are rendered practically useless if all one can do is move the knee back and forth a few degrees. In fact, a large part of your knee's functioning—probably more than most of us realize—depends quite heavily on its being flexible. A study done by Dr. Agustin Escalante and colleagues, of the University of Texas Health Science Center, demonstrated how essential a freely moving knee is to something as basic as walking. Working with a large study group of 702 subjects, he looked at many factors that might be associated with the speed at which people walk. Along with other variables, researchers recorded the motion of each participant's hip and knee joints, as well as how fast she or he could walk a distance of fifty feet. Interestingly, the study found that a subject's odds of being one of the slowest walkers increased up to six times by his or her having poor knee or hip flexibility. Apparently, the speed at which we walk depends greatly on how flexible our knees are.

A Little-Known Test of Knee Motion

At first glance, it would appear that all the knee joint does when we walk is merely swing back and forth, not unlike the hinge on a car door. The truth, however, is that your knee is also capable of rotating. That's right, rotating. With each step you or I take, the lower leg bone, the tibia, rotates outward. For those who find this a bit hard to visualize, try this simple demonstration:

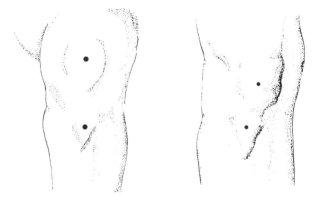

Figure 3.1 The right knee knee when it's bent   **Figure 3.2 The right when it's straightened**

Figure 3.1 illustrates what the knee looks like when you are in a sitting position, that is, when the knee is bent at about a ninety-degree angle. While sitting down, take a pen and place one mark in the middle of your kneecap (top dot) and one mark on the bony bump that sticks out on the lower leg just below your kneecap (bottom dot). Make sure you draw the dots in line with each other, as shown in Figure 3.1.

Next, while still sitting, kick your leg out. Your knee should now be straight and resemble Figure 3.2. Note that the dots are no longer in a straight line. This is because your lower leg bone rotated outward as you straightened your leg. This action also occurs when you are walking.

Pretty neat, huh? This nifty little test of knee motion is known as the *Helfet test*. Named after the orthopedic surgeon who developed it, Dr. Arthur Helfet, it has become a simple way of detecting rotation problems in the knee. If your knee is so tight that you are unable to do the test, don't get discouraged; stretching exercises can most certainly help you regain normal flexibility.

> ◆ *Your knee has three basic motions. It can bend backwards (flexion), straighten out (extension), and rotate.*
> ◆ *Stretching exercises can help restore all of these motions.*

Why Your Knee Isn't Flexible

Every reader will most likely experience a different amount of tightness in his or her knees. Some will be unable to fully straighten their knees, while others may have difficulty bending them. The specific stretches described in this chapter will help you to restore *all* the motions of your knee, getting it back to peak performance. But first, what is preventing your knee from moving freely?

Many reasons can exist for a lack of flexibility in the knees, and here again, no two readers may have the same exact cause. The following table lists some common conditions that can limit knee motion.

Problems that may lead to a loss of flexibility in the knee	Possible causes of this problem	Common treatments
Swelling	Fluid in the knee joint takes up space and prevents full motion	Ice, stretching, removal of fluid by needle, anti-inflammatory medications

Problems that may lead to a loss of flexibility in the knee	Possible causes of this problem	Common treatments
Tight muscles	Muscles become shorter when not regularly stretched through their full range	Stretching exercises
Mechanical problems	Problems such as torn cartilage or loose bodies in the joint can block normal motion between the bones	In some situations, surgical removal
Pain	A knee that hurts doesn't move through a full range of motion, causing muscles and other structures to shorten over time	Exercise, pain medications
Tight joint capsule	The tissue that surrounds the entire joint can become tight, keeping the bones from moving normally	Stretching, joint manipulation

You can see from the above list that there are various causes of lost knee motion—and, likewise, various treatments to correct these problems. Although this is a book on self-treatment, I would like to make it clear that not all cases can be treated conservatively at home. For instance, a person who has torn the cartilage in her or his knee—a problem that can mechanically block knee motion much like a marble in a gearbox—will quite possibly need surgery. Realistically, though, most people with this type of problem will probably not be reading this book, but rather will end up at the doctor's office, because it will be obvious that something major has gone wrong. Indeed, many readers with decreased knee motion can be more than adequately treated with a simple stretching program, done correctly. My only point here is to let you know that although stretching is indicated most frequently in the majority of cases, it is not a universal treatment. Please consult your medical professional should any questions arise.

Some readers may also have noticed that what is missing from the list of causes are specific ailments such as arthritis. That is because in this book we're more concerned with function rather than labels. Therefore, when looking at why a knee isn't bending, for instance, we don't say it's because of the arthritis, but rather because of the pain, swelling, or muscle tightness that's secondary to the arthritis. And why should we think about it like this? Because doing so helps us to better zero in on specific problems we can treat, as opposed to just blindly recommending that someone "slap a hot pack on their knee for twenty minutes and start walking more" because it's "good for arthritic knees."

◆ *Many things can limit knee motion.*
◆ *Stretching can help restore flexibility in many cases.*

Just How Much Motion Should a Normal Knee Have Anyway?

The range of motion a normal human knee is supposed to have depends very much on which source you happen to be consulting at the moment. Take a look at the following list I compiled from several different publications and you'll see what I mean:

Source	Normal amount of knee bending, in degrees
American Academy of Orthopedic Surgeons (1965)	135°
Clark (1920)	145°
Kapandji (1970)	160°
Journal of the American Medical Association (1958)	120°
Daniels and Worthingham (1972)	130°
Kendall and McCreary (1983)	140°

As with many questions, the answer seems to depend upon whom you talk to. If pushed into a corner, I'd have to say that the most commonly quoted number from most of the literature I've looked at is 135 degrees. This means that most people should be able to pull their heel back towards their rear end to an angle of 135 degrees. As for extension, the motion of straightening the leg, few would disagree that a normal knee should at least be able to straighten the leg all the way, making a perfectly straight line.

With all the apparent confusion over what's considered "normal," there is another way of approaching the whole issue. Rather than trying to increase our knee flexibility to a controversial "normal" range, maybe we should be more concerned with how much knee motion we actually need for our day-to-day activities and shoot for this as our personal standard.

Looking into this very matter, Dr. Phillip Rowe, of the Queen Margaret University College, and his colleagues conducted a very insightful study that determined exactly how much knee flexibility is necessary for us to be able to normally go about our daily business. Hooking up the knees of twenty healthy individuals to a fancy device called a *flexible electrogoniometer*, these researchers followed subjects around and recorded their knee motion as they performed eleven common activities. When all was said and done, here's what the study found:

Activity	Maximum amount of knee bending needed on average
Walking on level ground	67°
Walking up a 5° slope	65°
Walking down a 5° slope	72°
Climbing a twenty-step flight of stairs	99°
Going down a twenty-step flight of stairs	97°
Sitting down into a regular chair (about 18¼ inches high)	99°
Getting up from a regular chair	99°
Sitting down into a low chair (about 15 inches high)	102°
Getting up from a low chair	105°
Getting into the bathtub	131°

Readers with substantial losses of flexibility can use the above information to determine roughly how much range of motion they'll need in their knees for a particular activity, and this information will indicate how much flexibility they'll need to aim for with the stretching exercises. For instance, if you are having difficulty climbing stairs, the table tells us that your knees on average must be able to bend about 99 degrees to adequately perform that activity. To walk on level ground, your minimum goal would be about 67 degrees, and so on. Keep in mind that these are for *normal* daily activities. A reader who needs to function at a high level, such as an athlete—a hurdler, for example—probably needs the highest degree of knee motion that she or he can get.

When estimating how flexible your own knee is, use the 0-degree and 90-degree marks as points of reference. Zero degrees is a knee that is extended perfectly straight, while a knee bending at 90 degrees makes a right angle or "L" shape. From here, you can roughly estimate other points, such as 45 degrees (halfway between 0 and 90 degrees) or 135 degrees (halfway between 90 degrees and the back of the thigh).

> *When trying to figure out how flexible your knee will need to be, always take into account the specific activities that you do every day.*

Use These Stretching Secrets to Succeed

There are two secrets when it comes to successful stretching. The first is deciding exactly why you are stretching, and the second is making sure you are using guidelines that have been proven to work in research studies.

Let's first tackle the question "Why am I stretching?" This may seem like a ridiculous question until you know that there are two main reasons why people stretch:

◆ to temporarily decrease the tension in a muscle

◆ to permanently increase the length of a muscle

An example of the first case, to decrease tension in a muscle, would be stretching after you have been on a long car ride or sitting at a computer for a while. The muscles have become uncomfortable (rather than physically shortened) from being in one spot for too long and a stretch is clearly in order. So you get up, bend backwards or rotate your neck, and you feel much better. In these cases, stretching for a few seconds is clearly enough to accomplish the job.

The second case, stretching to permanently increase the length of a muscle, involves a whole different ball game. In this instance, a muscle is shorter in length than we want it to be, so we need to stretch it to actually increase its length over time. Here's where our second secret to stretching comes in: using guidelines that have been proven to work. (Note that the guidelines we will follow are entirely different from those we would follow for stretching to temporarily relieve built-up muscle tension.) The guidelines for stretching in order to permanently lengthen a muscle are as follows:

- If the muscle is contracted (severely shortened and tight) from being in one position for an extremely long period of time—such as in the case of a person who's been on bed rest for months, or an elbow that has been in a cast for six weeks—clinical studies tell us that what is usually needed is a low-load, prolonged stretch. An example of this would be putting a light weight around your wrist as you hang your arm, palm up, over the edge of a table for twenty minutes or so to stretch out your tight biceps muscle.

- If the muscle is tight and there has been no direct injury or trauma to it (such as surgery on the muscle itself), and it has not been stuck in one position for an extended period of time (such as a leg in traction for months), then clinical studies reveal that one stretch each day, held for thirty seconds and performed five days a week, is enough to cause the muscle to become longer over a period of just a few weeks.

Most readers who have tight muscles will in all probability fit into the second description and will require just one thirty-second stretch, one time a day, five days a week, to make their muscles longer and more flexible. These guidelines are taken directly from several published randomized controlled trials on stretching, where the investigators were trying to determine exactly how long a person needs to hold a stretch and how often they need to repeat it in order to gain the most flexibility (Bandy 1994, 1997). (Recall from the preceding chapter that randomized controlled trials are the highest form of proof in medicine that a treatment is truly effective.)

If, on the other hand, your muscles are extremely tight because your knee has been immobile for an extended period of time—say, for many weeks or months—then you will in all likelihood require a low-load, prolonged stretch to regain full knee mobility. If that is the case, I recommend seeing a medical professional, such as a physical therapist, as you will likely need supervision with these techniques, which are beyond the scope of this book. Also, since this book only covers knee treatments that you can safely do by yourself at home, please consult your doctor to treat other causes of poor knee flexibility (such as significant swelling) that you feel might be working against you.

> ◆ *If your muscles are tight, and if they have sustained no direct injury, surgery, or trauma, and if they have not been stuck in one position for an extended period of time (such as in a cast for two months), the research shows that one thirty-second stretch done once a day, five days a week, is sufficient to cause a muscle to lengthen over a period of weeks.*
>
> ◆ *If you have a contracted or severely shortened muscle due to its being in one position for a prolonged period of time (e.g., you were confined to bed rest or were in a cast for months), you will probably require a low-load, prolonged stretch to regain full flexibility in your knee. As these are usually not self-treatment techniques, please consult a medical professional.* (cont'd.)

> ◆ *There can be causes of decreased knee flexibility other than just tight muscles (e.g., substantial swelling), and these may require specific treatments. Again, talk with your doctor if you feel any of these situations might apply to you.*

It Only Takes Two Stretches to Get the Job Done

Okay, time now for the meat and potatoes of this chapter: the stretching exercises. There are two main muscle groups that we're most concerned about when it comes to restoring knee flexibility: the hamstrings and the quadriceps.

◆ **The hamstrings muscle group:** If you place your hand on the *back* of your thigh, you're right on these muscles. When tight, they keep your leg from straightening out all the way.

◆ **The quadriceps muscle group:** To feel these muscles, place your hand on the *front* of the thigh. If tight, they can keep you from being able to bend your leg back toward your buttocks.

To take into account the diverse abilities of many different readers (some may have difficulty standing up to do a stretch, while others may have trouble lying on their back), I have provided illustrations of how to stretch the hamstrings and quadriceps muscles in several different positions. Pick the stretch that is done in the position that is easiest for you.

HAMSTRING STRETCHES (PICK ONE)

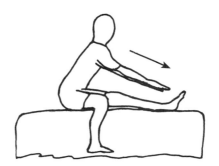

Figure 3.3 Hamstring stretch no. 1

- Get into the position shown in Figure 3.3, either on the floor or on a bed. Where you put your nonstretched leg makes no difference as long as it is in a comfortable spot.

- Lean forward toward your foot until a gentle stretch is felt in the *back* of your thigh. Try to bend forward from the hips as much as possible rather than bending from your back.

- Try to keep your knee straight.

- Hold this position for thirty seconds. Repeat on the other leg if you wish.

- Do the exercise once a day, five days a week, and gradually work up to thirty seconds if you have to.

By stretching in this manner, you are sending a signal to your muscle that it needs to elongate. Over a period of weeks, the muscle will gradually lengthen.

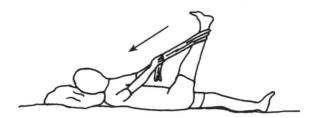

Figure 3.4 Hamstring stretch no. 2

- Using a towel, get into the position shown in Figure 3.4, either on the floor or on a bed.

- Pull your foot toward you until a gentle stretch is felt in the *back* of the thigh.

- Try to keep your knee straight.

- Hold this position for thirty seconds. Repeat on the other leg if you wish.

- Do the exercise once a day, five days a week, and gradually work up to thirty seconds if you have to.

By stretching in this manner, you are sending a signal to your muscle that it needs to elongate. Over a period of weeks, the muscle will gradually lengthen.

QUADRICEPS STRETCHES (PICK ONE)

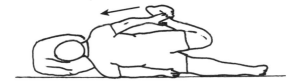

Figure 3.5 Quadriceps stretch no. 1

- Get into the position shown in Figure 3.5, either on the floor or on a bed.
- Grabbing your ankle, pull your foot backward toward your buttocks until you feel a gentle stretch in the *front* of your thigh.
- Bring your knee backward as well for an even stronger stretch.
- Hold this position for thirty seconds. Repeat on the other leg if you wish.
- Do the exercise once a day, five days a week. Work up to thirty seconds if you have to.

By stretching in this manner, you are sending a signal to your muscle that it needs to elongate. Over a period of weeks, the muscle will gradually lengthen.

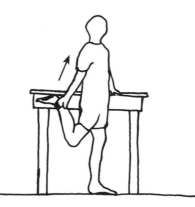

Figure 3.6 Quadriceps stretch no. 2

◆ Get into the position shown in Figure 3.6.

◆ Grabbing your ankle, pull your foot backward toward your buttocks until you feel a gentle stretch in the *front* of your thigh.

◆ Bring your knee backward as well for an even stronger stretch.

◆ Hold this position for thirty seconds. Repeat on the other leg if you wish.

◆ Do the exercise once a day, five days a week. Work up to thirty seconds if you have to.

By stretching in this manner, you are sending a signal to your muscle that it needs to elongate. Over a period of weeks, the muscle will gradually lengthen.

Pretty simple, huh? If you use the guidelines provided, stretching to lengthen the muscles that provide mobility to your knee doesn't have to be an all-day affair. Also, remember to pick only one stretch for your hamstrings muscle group and one stretch for your quadriceps. Therefore, you should be doing a grand total of only two stretches a day, taking you sixty seconds to complete (thirty seconds per exercise), push down a minimal investment of your time in an activity that is going to give you a much more efficient knee—and in turn a lot less pain!

4

Improving Your Proprioception

Although the word proprioception may look confusing, all this fourteen-letter word means is the ability you have at any given moment to sense the position and movements of your body. For instance, as you are reading this book, you could probably tell me without difficulty if your legs are bent or straight, crossed or uncrossed, all without even looking. To give you more of an idea of just how useful proprioception is, here are a few everyday activities whose success or failure depends heavily on the proper functioning of your sense of proprioception:

- getting keys out of your pocket
- scratching that hard-to-reach spot on your back
- pushing down on the gas or brake pedal in your car
- walking to the bathroom in the middle of the night without falling

As you may have noticed, all of these particular activities involve getting something done without the help of your vision. By giving your brain constant updates as to the position of your arms and legs, your proprioception is most able to help you when you are unable to see exactly what you are doing.

Another good example of how crucial the sense of proprioception is to our day-to-day existence comes from a patient I had who lacked proprioception in both of his legs. Unfortunately, this gentleman suffered from a condition called *CIDP,* or *chronic inflammatory demyelinating polyneuropathy*, a rare neurological disorder involving destruction of the covering around the nerves. As his physical therapist, my job was to get him out of the bed and see how well he could walk.

The first hurdle we had to cross, getting him onto his feet, proved to be somewhat easy; we used a walker and his legs were quite strong. Walking, however, turned out to be another matter entirely. Each step was a journey into the unknown. Since his legs gave him little feedback as to where they actually were, his whole leg would begin to swing wildly in a circular motion as he desperately tried to place his foot on the floor. Even though he knew where he wanted his legs to go and had plenty of strength to make them move, it was impractical for him to walk any meaningful distance without proprioception.

A Knee Without Proprioception Could Be Headed for Trouble

As you can see, there is much we would be unable do without our sense of proprioception. Most readers of this book, however, will be in nowhere near the kind of shape my patient was in. Having proprioception problems to the degree he suffered usually occurs when one has a serious problem with her or his nervous system. Perhaps that is why proprioception exercises are usually either last on the list of treatments for knee pain or are neglected entirely. A lot of medical professionals tend to think of proprioception problems as happening only in patients with grave neurological disorders. Nothing, as you will soon see, could be further from the truth; plenty of research studies have shown many types of knee conditions to be associated with abnormal proprioception.

Most proprioception problems in the knee arise from conditions such as arthritis or injury, and these tend to be less severe than those stemming from serious nervous-system problems. However, they still deserve attention and treatment. Although your proprioception may be only slightly impaired, you should be aware that *any* decrease in your knee's ability to sense position and movement can put your knee at risk for injury or damage. Here's one such example. Say you're merrily walking along with a friend and are temporarily distracted as you're talking. Suddenly, you happen to step off a curb you didn't know was there. This catches you off guard and sends a sudden "jolt" throughout your entire leg and knee joint. What happens next depends to a large degree on how well your proprioception works. Consider the following:

◆ The knee with *normal* proprioception can send information to the brain about your leg's position and movements in a split second. In turn, the leg muscles can react immediately by contracting to maintain your balance and posture, as well as by stabilizing your knee to keep it in a safe position.

◆ The knee with *decreased* proprioception fails to react nearly as fast and therefore puts your knee at risk for injury (as well as putting you at risk for falling down).

The lesson in all this is that proprioception very much serves a protective role. When the nerves in your leg muscles, tendons, and joint capsules immediately send feedback to your brain as to what's going on, you can quickly get things under control and avoid a knee injury or worse. This line of thinking is just now beginning to catch on, and it has been proven to work successfully with athletes. In one of the most scientifically advanced studies to date on the protective role of proprioception training on the knee, four orthopedic surgeons studied a whopping nine hundred European soccer players and found that exercises to improve proprioception and balance actually *prevented* future knee injuries compared to the control group (Caraffa 1996).

> *Proprioception helps to protect your knee from injury and joint damage.*

If You're on this List, Your Knee Could Have Proprioception Problems

Up to now we've established that most proprioception problems in the knee, while not on the severe end of the scale, are nonetheless significant *and* can possibly set up the knee for an injury. Some readers may be wondering to what degree proprioception is typically impaired in people with knee problems. Many studies have tested proprioception in people with various knee conditions and have consistently noted subtle yet important changes.

Let's look at how such studies test proprioception. A researcher in a study might take someone with, say, knee arthritis and do the following test:

- ◆ The subject's knees are hooked up to a sophisticated device that reliably measures the angle at which the knee is bent.

- ◆ The subject closes his or her eyes.

- ◆ The test starts with the subject's knee in a standard straight position.

- ◆ The researcher bends the subject's knee to a certain angle, holds it briefly, and then returns it to the straight position.

◆ The subject is asked if he or she can bend the knee to exactly the same angle as the researcher did.

What the researchers usually find is that while most subjects usually have enough proprioception to walk around and "know" where their legs are, they actually perform very poorly in "picky" tests, such as the one described above.

The next question that probably pops into your mind is exactly who with knee problems might have trouble with proprioception. To answer that question, I did what I always do: I read what the research has to say about the matter. After reviewing all the studies I could get my hands on about proprioception testing of the knee, I compiled a list of several types of knee conditions that have been shown to be associated with decreased proprioception. The list is as follows:

◆ people with patellofemoral pain syndrome (pain felt behind or around the knee)

◆ people with knee osteoarthritis

◆ people who have ruptured their anterior cruciate ligament

◆ people who have dislocated their kneecap

◆ people over sixty years of age

◆ people who have torn their medial meniscus

Some readers may find themselves on the list and others may not. At this point, I want you to do the following:

◆ If you *do* think you fit into one of the above descriptions, there is a good chance that you might have a problem with proprioception, in which case you will greatly benefit from the proprioception exercises.

◆ If you *don't* think you fit any into any of the above descriptions, I want you to try the proprioception exercises anyway. If you can do them correctly, your proprioception is probably adequate. If, on the other hand, you find you cannot do them properly, you should add them to your list of knee exercises to perform.

Many studies have shown that people with knee pain and various knee injuries have problems with proprioception.

A Simple Way to Work On Improving Your Proprioception

Of all the exercises that I recommend in this book, this one is the most straightforward and requires the least amount of equipment. In fact, all it involves is standing on one leg!

Once you read through the exercises described below, and before you embrace the notion that they are too easy, try them out. I think you'll find them more challenging than they sound. By practicing balancing on one leg for a period of time, you will be causing the following several things to occur in your knee:

◆ Your knee joint will be bearing weight, which will stimulate the nerves involved in proprioception, "exercising" them, if you will.

◆ The leg muscles will get good practice in stabilizing the knee joint.

Once you tackle standing on one leg, the next step will be for you to stand on one leg *with your eyes closed*. Without being able to see, you will have to rely even more on your sense of proprioception to stand on one leg, which will work your proprioception even harder. Now let's take a closer look at the exercises.

PROPRIOCEPTION EXERCISE NO. 1: EYES OPEN

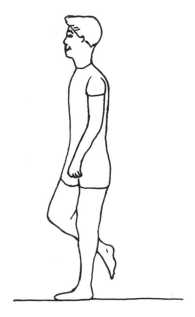

Figure 4.1 Proprioception exercise

- Stand on one leg in the same position as illustrated in Figure 4.1. The knee can be straight or slightly bent, whichever is more comfortable.

- If you can't stand on one leg at all, *or* if you can but you're really off balance and might fall, you can stand next to a table, chair, or doorway—something you can lightly hold on to.

- Repeat the exercise on the other leg if you wish.

- When you can stand well balanced on either leg for thirty full seconds, without holding on to anything, move on to exercise no. 2.

PROPRIOCEPTION EXERCISE NO. 2: EYES CLOSED

- ◆ Stand on one leg in the same position as illustrated in Figure 4.1. This time, keep both eyes closed. The knee can be straight or slightly bent, whichever is more comfortable.

- ◆ If you can't stand on one leg at all, *or* if you can but you're really off balance and might fall, you can stand next to a table, chair, or doorway—something you can lightly hold on to.

- ◆ Repeat the exercise on the other leg if you wish.

- ◆ When you can stand well balanced on either leg for thirty full seconds, without holding on to anything and with your eyes closed, your proprioception should be in much better shape.

Although these exercises may seem ridiculously simple, I think most readers will find them a bit more challenging than they look. Since there is little research telling us how often a person needs to do these exercise to get *the best* results, I recommend doing them three times a week with a day of rest in between, just as with the strengthening exercise for the quadriceps. Week by week, the exercises will begin to get easier and easier, indicating that you're well on your way to improving your proprioception.

5

Simple Ways to Increase Your Knee Endurance

I've always been amazed by the extreme limits to which a human body can be pushed when someone puts their mind to doing something. According to the *Guinness Book of World Records*, some of the most amazing achievements of human determination include the following:

- tap dancing a distance of 32 miles in 7 hours and 35 minutes

- balancing on one foot for 76 hours and 40 minutes

- running on a treadmill for 24 hours straight while covering a distance of 93.5 miles

- blowing up and tying 599 balloons in one hour

- swimming 122 miles in the ocean in 38 hours and 33 minutes

- jumping on a pogo stick for 23.22 miles in 12 hours and 27 minutes

- kissing for 30 hours and 45 minutes

- clapping continuously for 58 hours and 9 minutes, while maintaining an average of 160 claps per minute

Notice that all of these astounding feats have a common thread running through them: None of them could have been accomplished without the one ability that also happens to be the topic of this chapter—endurance. As you might gather, endurance is absolutely essential to your knee if it is going to be able to do anything required of it for a sustained period of time.

Why Knee Pain Can Spell Double Trouble for Your Endurance

This chapter is concerned with restoring the ability of endurance to your knee. But what exactly do we mean by *endurance*? Most people would say it's the ability to do something over and over for a long period of time. That's true. However, when discussing your knee and endurance, we need to get a bit more specific.

Among the many hair-pulling classes I took in physical-therapy school, my physiology class probably dealt with the topic of endurance in the most detail. I learned that as far as the human body is concerned, there are two basic types of endurance:

1. *Cardiovascular endurance*, or as I like to call it, "whole body" endurance. This is the ability your body has to do something over and over again, usually involving several large muscle groups. Walking for two full hours is one such example. It involves repeated contractions in just about all the muscles of your legs, and it works your heart as well.

2. *Muscular endurance*. This is the ability of a single muscle or muscle group to contract repeatedly. An example of this would be sitting in a chair and kicking your right leg out continuously for ten minutes. Unlike walking or running, which involves many muscle groups and body parts, doing this would be an endurance event involving mainly just your quadriceps muscle group.

What is the point of this discussion? We need to differentiate between the two types of endurance so we know exactly what we're talking about when discussing endurance problems in people who suffer knee pain. Knee pain, unlike other problems such as shoulder or neck pain, affects more than just the endurance of your individual knee muscles (such as the quadriceps group). Because it also affects your ability to get up and go, it often takes its toll on your overall cardiovascular endurance as well. Therefore, in order to get you fully up to par again, we need to be sure that we treat both kinds of endurance.

> *Knee pain not only has a tendency to limit the endurance of the individual muscles around the knee, but it can also affect your overall cardiovascular endurance as well.*

In Five Minutes, You're Going to Know the Basics of Knee Endurance

Yes, it's true. Five minutes from now (providing you read at a reasonable pace) you will know the basics of endurance. Don't panic—I'm not going to try to turn you into an exercise physiologist. I just want you to have a little knowledge of how endurance is made possible so you'll understand more clearly how we're going to restore it.

Ready? First lesson: It takes energy to run your body. (I told you I wasn't going to get technical.) Second lesson: As long as you keep supplying the body with energy, it will keep going. Run out of energy and things will start to slow down and eventually come to a grinding halt. The big question, then, is how do our bodies and muscles get a constant supply of energy to keep them working?

In order to meet the demands of daily living, your body relies on the following three "energy systems":

- ◆ the phosphagen system
- ◆ the glycogen–lactic acid system
- ◆ the aerobic system

You don't have to remember the names of the three energy systems or even know how to pronounce them. Just know that there are three of them.

The next key piece of information is that each of these energy systems supplies energy to your muscles at different times during a particular activity. Allow me to clarify this by having you perform the following test (you can just read it if you prefer). All you need is a wristwatch and a foot.

- ◆ Start timing yourself and begin tapping your foot up and down on the floor continuously.

- ◆ During the first ten seconds of tapping, the muscles you use get their energy mainly from the phosphagen energy system. Unfortunately, this system only supplies energy for about ten seconds.

- ◆ Keep tapping. From the ten-second mark up to around the two-minute mark, the muscles you use mainly get their energy from the glycogen–lactic acid energy system. This particular system kicks in only after you've been doing something for around ten seconds. Unfortunately, it fizzles out after about two minutes.

- ◆ If you keep tapping longer than two minutes, the muscles you use get their energy from the aerobic energy system. This system only gets cranked up after you've been doing an activity for more than about two minutes, and it becomes the major provider of energy from this point on.

Okay, time to give that foot a rest. As you can see, the body uses the three energy systems in a certain order, with each one supplying energy at certain points during an activity. Here's another way of looking at the whole process:

System	Time frame
Phosphagen system	Supplies energy for about the first 8–10 seconds of an activity
Glycogen–lactic acid system	Starts supplying energy after the first 10 seconds or so of an activity and continues up to around 2 minutes
Aerobic system	Kicks in after you do an activity for longer than about 2 minutes and continues to supply the energy for the activity until you quit

One of the best analogies I've heard used to describe the three energy systems is to compare them to the gears in a car. You always start out in first gear (the phosphagen system) but quickly find that you can't travel for very long in that gear. So you shift to second gear (the glycogen–lactic acid system), which takes you a bit farther, but not quite up to cruising speed. To be able to cruise, you need to shift into third gear (the aerobic system), which is a gear that allows you to maintain your speed for the rest of the trip.

Now that you have a basic idea of the way your body keeps you fueled with energy, how are we going to use the information? First of all, let me say that the more you use a particular energy system, the more efficient the system becomes. For instance, power lifters, who lift huge weights over a few seconds, tend to use only the first energy system, the phosphagen system, and so it becomes more efficient. On the other hand, marathon runners, who literally run for hours, have highly developed aerobic energy systems, simply because they use and tax that particular energy system the most. In a nutshell, remember that the more a particular energy system gets worked, the more efficient that system will become.

When we apply this knowledge to an effort to increase the endurance of the knee, we must first consider the kinds of activities the knee will be doing each day, and what energy system it will be using the most. For a lot of readers, their knees will be involved in normal daily activities, such as walking or standing, activities that require them to work for more than two minutes at a time. Therefore, we must set our sights on training the aerobic energy system to get better at doing these kinds of prolonged activities and to do them more efficiently. This is exactly what the exercises at the end of this chapter are designed to do: restore the ability of endurance to your knee by working the aerobic energy system using a simple exercise.

> ◆ *Your body uses three energy systems to keep it supplied with energy.*
> ◆ *The more you use a particular energy system, the more efficient it will become.*

Two More Reasons Why Your Knee Needs Good Muscular Endurance

For four years I worked on a busy orthopedic floor in a large teaching hospital. Every week or two, like clockwork, an older patient would be admitted to the floor after falling and fracturing a bone. More often than not, a hipbone had been broken and the poor patient would inevitably have to undergo some type of surgery. The orthopedic surgeons, greatly skilled in fixing bones, could usually repair the break through the use of plates and screws. In some cases, however, when a patient was unlucky enough to have broken a bone that significantly damaged the blood supply to the joint, a total hip replacement usually followed.

There are, of course, lots of reasons why people fall. After reading a 1997 study conducted by the University of Indiana School of Medicine, I believe we can add muscular endurance to the list.

This novel study investigated three different groups of women: a young group, an older group with a history of falling, and an older group without a history of falling. (The older women were around seventy and the younger women were around twenty.) Data were collected on the subjects, including examination of the muscular endurance of each woman's quadriceps muscle and how fast it could recover after a bout of exercise. Here's what the results on muscular endurance revealed:

◆ Those with a history of falling had much worse muscular endurance than those without a history of falling.

◆ Muscular endurance was not different between the older women without a history of falling and the younger women.

Most readers might have guessed that the fallers would have far less muscular endurance in their quadriceps muscles than the non-fallers. However, it probably came as a surprise to many that the older non-fallers had basically the same amount of muscular endurance as the younger women! According to these results, as you get older, you don't automatically lose your muscular endurance, but if you do, it can definitely put you at risk for falling.

Another interesting study, this one specifically concerning muscular endurance and knee pain, was reported in a 1991 article published in *Medicine and Science in Sports and Exercise*. Dr. Messier and colleagues at Wake Forest University investigated several factors that might be associated with patellofemoral pain in runners. *Patella* is the medical term for the kneecap; *femoral* refers to the femur or thigh bone. Therefore, in layman's terms, patello-femoral pain is knee pain that is behind or around the kneecap.

The researchers compared sixteen runners diagnosed with patellofemoral pain to a control group of twenty healthy runners. Once again, differences in muscular endurance stood out between the two groups. More interesting than that, however, was the fact that muscular endurance was found to be an important predictor of who did and did not have knee pain. The following are few details from the study:

◆ Runners with knee pain showed decreased muscular endurance, especially in the quadriceps muscle group (no surprise).

◆ If you took both groups in the study—i.e., those with and those without knee pain—and mixed them together in one room, you could correctly place 92 percent of the healthy control subjects and 80 percent of the knee-pain subjects into their respective groups based solely upon muscular-endurance variables.

Don't you think it's interesting that one could actually predict 80 percent of the runners who suffered knee pain simply based on the poor endurance capabilities of their knee muscles? Clearly, muscular endurance is not the only factor involved in a person's knee pain, but studies like this one certainly make one think twice about how important it is to have a knee with good muscular endurance.

> *Poor endurance of the knee muscles has been associated not only with knee pain, but with other things as well, such as an increased risk of falling in the elderly.*

Four Exercises to Increase Knee Endurance

Hopefully by this point I've sold you on the importance of having a knee with good endurance—that is, a knee with the ability to do its job over and over again. Now I'm going to show you how to get it. The following exercises are four of the best and easiest ways for you to increase the endurance of your knee muscles. Since these activities involve the repetitive contraction of large muscles, such as your quadriceps, your heart and cardiovascular system will get a workout as well. That's why it's really important that your doctor give you the okay before you undertake the exercises in this book.

Having said that, here are the endurance exercises. You will need to do only one of them to increase your endurance, so pick the one you like best. You can also alternate among them or switch periodically to avoid becoming bored.

ENDURANCE EXERCISE NO. 1

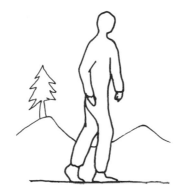

Figure 5.1 Endurance exercise No. 1

Yes, the first endurance exercise is simply walking. It's uncomplicated, gets the job done, and requires only space. But you do have to follow a few rules in order to get the endurance benefits we're looking for.

■◆ Walk at a pace that is comfortable for you. The key here is that while it doesn't really matter how fast you are walking, you must keep moving continuously in order to build endurance.

◆ Go for time, not distance. Your goal is to work up to twenty or thirty minutes of continuous walking, two or three times a week. Whether you start by walking for one minute or for ten minutes doesn't matter. Let's say you can only walk for eight minutes the first time. Next time, try to walk for nine or ten minutes. With each session, try to increase the time that you walk by a little bit. By doing so in a progressive manner, you'll soon be walking the full twenty or thirty minutes.

- Tips: I suggest walking in supportive athletic shoes or shoes designed specifically for walking. Also wear cushioned athletic socks and loose-fitting clothing. If balance is an issue, use the appropriate assistive device (e.g. cane, walker, friend) to stay safe.

ENDURANCE EXERCISE NO. 2

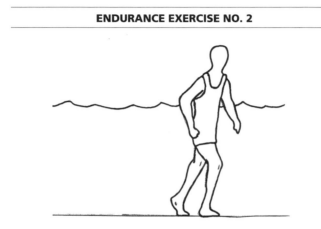

Figure 5.2 Endurance exercise No. 2

Walking in a pool is the second endurance exercise. Because the water helps to support your body, walking in water offers the advantage of exercising your knee without placing the whole weight of your body upon it.

- Use the same guidelines for pool walking as you do for walking on land. Walk at a comfortable pace, try to keep moving continuously, do two or three sessions a week, and eventually work up to twenty or thirty minutes total per session. Do this by progressively adding a minute or two at each session.

- You can adjust the amount of resistance you experience by changing your depth in the water:

- With the water up to your neck, you're at approximately 10% of your true body weight

- With the water up to your chest, you're at approximately 25% of your true body weight

- With the water up to your waist, you're at approximately 50% of your true body weight

◆ Tips: Never exercise alone in the water. You may wish to wear aquatic shoes to protect and cushion your feet.

ENDURANCE EXERCISE NO. 3

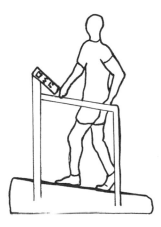

Figure 5.3 Endurance exercise No. 3

Endurance exercise number three involves walking on a treadmill. It is similar to walking on land except that you are forced to keep walking at a certain pace. This is because the belt under your feet keeps moving at a fixed pace, requiring you to go as fast as the treadmill does. Therefore, if you choose to do this exercise, set the treadmill at a pace that you are comfortable with!

- ◆ Start out with the treadmill flat.

- ◆ Whether you hold on to the side rails or let your hands swing freely depends entirely upon how good your balance is. This is where you have to be the judge. Remember, safety first.

- ◆ Set the treadmill to a comfortable speed.

- ◆ Go for time. Try to eventually work up to a total of twenty or thirty minutes total by progressively adding a minute or two at each session. Do two or three sessions a week.

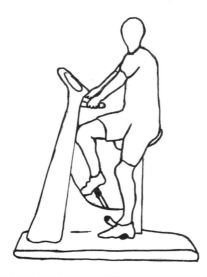

ENDURANCE EXERCISE NO. 4

Figure 5.4 Endurance exercise No. 4

The last endurance exercise you can choose is using a stationary exercise bike. Like water walking, using an exercise bike is advantageous because it works your knee without you having to place the weight of your body on your knee.

◆ Don't just hop on an exercise bike and start pedaling. Seat height is very important. A seat that is too low will cause your knee to bend too much and can actually create additional problems. A seat that is too high is less hard on your knee but can be very uncomfortable because it leaves you "reaching" for the pedal. Be aware of seat height, and, above all, set it so your knee is comfortable while pedaling all the way through the pedal cycle. Long-distance bicyclists often cycle for hours at a time, so they're very tuned into what's comfortable and what isn't. Consider using the same guideline for seat height that they use. They adjust the seat so that when the pedal is at the bottom of the revolution there is a very slight bend in the knee.

◆ Set the bike on the least amount of resistance.

◆ Go for time. Try to eventually work up to twenty or thirty minutes per session by progressively adding a minute or two at each session. Do two or three sessions a week.

6

Some Things You May *Not* Have Thought About

As the story goes, an elderly gentleman went to visit his doctor, complaining that he had trouble getting around because of a terrible pain in his right knee. After a careful examination, the doctor turned to the man and said, "It's probably just old age. You know you are seventy years old." Looking a bit puzzled, the patient paused for a second and then replied, "Well, my left knee is just as old and it doesn't hurt."

While amusing and funny, the story succeeds in making a very important point. Because the doctor finds nothing unusual after examining the patient's knee, he chalks it up to arthritis, given the man's old age. This is a logical assumption and it might indeed actually be the case. You'll note, however, that I said *might*. As the elderly gentleman is quick to point out, the other knee is just as old as the painful one and more than likely has undergone similar arthritic changes throughout the years, and yet it isn't bothersome at all. If arthritis really is the culprit, then why is only one knee affected?

As you will see in the pages that follow, it is far from an open-and-shut case that structural abnormalities such as worn-down knee cartilage, bony spurs, or a torn meniscus *always* cause knee pain. Quite to the contrary, many studies show the complete opposite: people walking around with structural abnormalities in their knees and yet have no pain whatsoever.

On my journeys through the medical research, I have found, sometimes by accident, much good research published in respected, peer-reviewed journals that has rigorously documented such instances. So interesting and thought-provoking did I find this research that I felt a book on knee pain without mention of it could not be considered complete. In this chapter, we will take a pit stop from looking at knee pain from the usual structural point of view and instead take a brief look at other things that might enter into the bigger picture of your knee pain; in particular, we will look at psychological factors. While this may sound a bit rebellious, I have only to prove to you that psychological factors can have just as much to do with knee pain as can a knee that has run out of cartilage.

Why Is Knee Arthritis So Frequently Pain-Free?

Starting in 1948, a group of more than five thousand adult residents from the small Massachusetts town of Framingham agreed to participate in an ongoing study that required them to undergo a very detailed examination every two years, including laboratory tests, chest X rays, and electrocardiograms. Known as the Framingham Heart Study, this mammoth study was originally undertaken to track a large population of people over a long period of time in order to better understand how heart disease, the number-one cause of death in the United States, develops. The study is now considered to be one of the most important in the annals of medical history, mainly because the vast majority of information we have today about important risk factors for heart disease, such as high blood pressure and elevated cholesterol, were a mystery before this study took place. In fact, before the Framingham Heart Study, many doctors believed that a person's blood pressure was supposed to naturally increase as the person aged, in order to allow the heart to pump blood more easily through clogged arteries.

In the early eighties, a group of clever researchers decided to take advantage of the Framingham Heart Study participants' biannual checkup to gain more knowledge about the occurrence of knee arthritis in the elderly. In a study published in the academic journal *Arthritis and Rheumatism*, Dr. David Felson and coworkers took knee X rays of 1,424 subjects whose ages ranged from sixty-three to ninety-four, exactly the time in life when one would expect knee arthritis to rear its ugly head. In addition to the X rays, a physical examination of the knee was performed and information was gathered about the amount of knee pain each person experienced.

Knee arthritis was graded on a commonly used scale of 0 to 4, with 0 meaning that no arthritic changes were visible on the knee X ray, and 4 designating the most severe arthritis. When the researchers finished crunching the numbers at the end of the study, here's what they found:

- ◆ 11 percent of the subjects who were between the ages of sixty-five and sixty-nine had grade-3 or grade-4 knee arthritis;

- ◆ 25 percent of the subjects who were eighty-five or older had grade-3 or grade-4 arthritis;

- ◆ only 40 percent of all subjects whose X rays indicated grade-3 or grade-4 arthritis experienced symptoms.

Wow. Let's ponder these results for a minute. It seems that the older a subject was, the more knee arthritis was seen on the X ray, which makes sense. More unexpected, though, was the fact that only a mere 40 percent of those with the most severe arthritic changes had symptoms, leaving the remaining 60 percent without pain!

How can this be? Were the results just a fluke, or an example of poor research? No, it appears not. Indeed, many other studies have found very similar results. Here are a couple more examples published in academic journals:

- In a study of 1,198 subjects, only 56 percent of men with grade-3 or grade-4 knee arthritis (the most severe) had any pain. For the women who had grade-3 or grade-4 knee arthritis, 80 percent reported pain (Lawrence 1966).

- Another study X-rayed 84 seventy-nine-year-olds and 76 eighty-five-year-olds and found that only 43 percent of those subjects with grade-3 or grade-4 knee arthritis had any pain complaints (Bagge 1991).

As the research is clearly telling us, it is far from a given that *all* knees with severe arthritis give rise to pain. Indeed, there are many individuals who have considerable X-ray evidence of disease in their knee, but who oddly experience a complete absence of symptoms.

So what about those people who have severe knee arthritis and who *are* in a lot of pain? What will happen to them over time? Are they destined to a life of pain until the inevitable day comes when they must hobble before a surgeon to get relief? Let's do what we always do for some answers and see what the research has to say. I know of two good studies that have helped shed some light on this area. The most recent one was presented at the 2002 Annual European Congress of Rheumatology. This study set out to investigate whether any link existed over a prolonged period of time between a person's progressively deteriorating arthritic knee and commonly experienced symptoms, such as pain, stiffness, and decreased mobility.

One hundred and six patients with knee arthritis were followed for three years. X rays of their knees were taken before and after the study and were used to measure the joint space—that is, the distance between the two bones (the tibia and femur) that make up the knee joint. Measuring joint space in the knee can indicate how much wear on the knee cartilage has occurred. This is because as the cartilage wears down, the two bones move closer together, resulting in a smaller space between the bones, as seen on the X-ray picture. Here is what the investigators found:

◆ No connection could be found between more narrowing of the joint space and worsening knee pain over time.

◆ No significant link existed between more narrowing of the joint space and a subject's ability to function.

The second study that tracked arthritic knees over time to see how closely progressive structural damage was tied to worsening of symptoms was published in the prestigious *Annals of the Rheumatic Diseases*. This time, researchers followed thirty-one patients with established, symptomatic knee arthritis over an eight-year time frame. Here are some interesting findings:

◆ Seven patients remained the same over the eight-year period.

◆ Twenty patients got worse.

◆ Four patients actually experienced improved knee symptoms, despite the fact that three of the four patients actually lost knee motion and developed more severe arthritic changes on their X rays over the eight-year study period.

◆ Changes seen in symptoms, disability, and X rays did not correlate at all.

The main theme of all this research seems to be that it is quite common for our knees to look worse and worse on an X ray as we get older. Despite these aging changes, however, what is not inevitable, as all five studies point out, is a life of pain and disability.

> ◆ *Multiple studies have demonstrated that there are many people who have severe arthritic changes in their knees as shown on an X ray and yet who have* no pain.
>
> ◆ *Arthritic knees can keep structurally deteriorating as time goes on, but this does not mean the pain will get worse. In fact, some studies show that people actually improve over time despite their knees looking worse on X rays.*
>
> ◆ *According to the available research, there is little association between knee pain, disability, and how a person's knee looks on an X ray.*

Do You Have Any "Normal" Abnormal Findings in Your Knee?

After reading these studies showing that many people actually have a structurally deteriorating knee and yet experience few symptoms, I started to rethink things. Of course, structural problems such as the loss of cartilage or the resulting overgrowth of bone can most certainly cause pain. But as the literature points out, these changes are a common, if not a natural, part of the aging process and definitely do not *always* cause pain. So, I wondered, what should I call such findings when I come across them in my patients? What to label findings that while technically "abnormal" are still quite common, yet cause the patient no problems?

After much thought, I decided to refer to these types of findings as "normal" abnormal. The label seemed to make sense, especially in the case of arthritis. An arthritic joint, while clearly showing changes from what is considered "normal," could at the same time be considered a normal part of the aging process, and, hence, the arthritis is a "normal" abnormal finding. The next mission I set for myself was to find out how many other "normal" abnormal findings might be found in the knee—that is, conditions considered abnormal in that they are clearly different from a normal knee, yet that are nonetheless very common and don't always cause pain. The results of my research were eye opening. Here's a sample:

- In 1989, Brunner et al., using an MRI, examined the knees of twenty athletes with no knee symptoms. Fifty percent of them showed abnormalities, which included abnormally appearing knee meniscus, posterior cruciate ligaments, and medial collateral ligaments.

- In 1990, Kornick et al. used an MRI to examine the pain-free knees of sixty-four volunteers ages ten to seventy-four. They found a 25 percent prevalence of knee meniscus abnormalities as early as the second decade of life; the incidence increased sharply with age.

- In 1991, Shellock performed an MRI on the pain-free knees of twenty-three marathon runners and found that 9 percent of them had meniscal tears and 45 percent had meniscal degeneration.

- In 1992, Boden et al. scanned the knees of seventy-four symptom-free volunteers with an MRI. Sixteen percent of the subjects had a meniscal tear, 7 percent showed moderate joint swelling, and 8 percent had a popliteal cyst (located behind the knee joint).

In the previous section, we looked at studies that used X rays to examine subjects' knees. The use of X ray is one of the best ways to see bony changes that have occurred in the knee. In this section we looked at studies that used MRI to examine the knee. MRI is better than X rays for observing changes in the soft tissues, such as ligaments and cartilage. As you can see, a similar theme keeps popping up among the various studies, whether they used X ray or MRI. Many structures in the knee can develop conditions considered "abnormal" and yet may cause no pain. Note that I am not saying that these structural abnormalities will never cause pain, but rather that a person can have some of these structural abnormalities and live just fine with them. When this occurs, I prefer to call it a "normal" abnormal finding.

◆ *If you know that your knee has a structural abnormality, do not be so quick to pin your knee pain on the abnormality. It may simply be what I call a "normal" abnormal finding. A structural finding is significant if it correlates well with the signs and symptoms you are having, which can be determined with the help of a medical professional.*

◆ *Since many structural knee abnormalities are common, it is hard to determine the true cause of knee pain in a lot of cases. This is the beauty of the approach I use in this book of treating your knee function rather than a specific cause or diagnosis; it bypasses the whole guessing game of what the true cause really is and will most likely help you get better!*

A Picture Is *Not* Worth a Thousand Words When It Comes to Your Knee

Up to now, we have taken a peek at some of the studies on knee arthritis that demonstrate that as we get older, it is normal for our knees to show variable rates of wear and tear on an X-ray picture. Although logic would dictate that a worn joint must surely cause debilitating knee pain, these studies have surprisingly pointed out that only *some* people with severe structural changes in their knee experience pain, while a great many others somehow escape symptoms. The next question to ask is whether there are other factors associated with knee pain besides purely structural changes in the knee.

To find answers to this question, studies have usually examined a group of people with knee arthritis for combinations of the following variables:

- level of disability or functional impairment
- intensity of knee pain
- X-ray pictures of subjects' knees
- psychosocial factors such as personality, life stress, anxiety, or depression

Let's talk a bit more about that last category, psychosocial factors. As soon as the studies began to flood the literature showing that a person could have various structural abnormalities in the knee without experiencing a whimper of pain, researchers began in particular to explore the psychological side of the person with knee pain. After all, if structural abnormalities weren't always the culprit, and people were living just fine with degenerating joints and torn knee cartilage, what else was left but the mind? When one delves into the knee literature, one notices an abundance of research concerning psychological factors and the patient with knee pain. Since the condition of knee arthritis is so common and causes the worst structural changes of all the knee-pain culprits, most of these studies were done on people with knee arthritis.

After gathering information about the variables involved in knee pain, researchers can scientifically look for any associations that might exist between a structurally deteriorating knee and pain and disability. The following is a synopsis of a few major studies that have succeeded in doing so:

◆ In 1988, Summers et al. studied sixty-five patients ages fifty-five to eighty-seven with hip and/or knee arthritis. X rays, psychological variables (depression, anxiety, coping style), functional impairment, and pain were all assessed. Surprisingly, the severity of one's arthritis showed little relationship to pain. On the other hand, the psychological variables were strong predictors of both functional impairment and pain.

◆ In 1991, Salaffi et al. examined sixty-one women ages fifty-one to seventy-nine with knee arthritis. X rays, amount of disability, anxiety, depression, and pain were all assessed. Results showed that the level of disability a subject experienced was more related to age and psychological variables than to how bad her knee arthritis looked on the X ray. Both anxiety and depression rose as important predictors of pain.

◆ In 1993, McAlindon et al. looked at seventy men and eighty-nine women over the age of fifty-five to try to determine how the functional ability of patients with knee arthritis was influenced by quadriceps strength, degree of arthritis seen on X ray, gender, and age. They found that quadriceps strength, knee pain, and age had much more to do with the level of functional impairment a person with knee arthritis suffered than did the severity of the arthritis seen on an X-ray picture.

◆ In 1998, VanBaar et al. conducted a study to determine what factors contributed the most to pain and disability in two hundred patients with hip or knee arthritis. They looked quite extensively at many variables: pain, level of disability, X rays, muscle strength, joint range of motion, pain coping ability, depression, anxiety, and cheerfulness. Interestingly, pain was associated with muscle weakness and coping ability. Disability was associated with muscle weakness, joint range of motion, pain, pain coping ability, and psychological well-being. How the subject's joint looked on the X-ray picture was not significantly associated with pain or disability.

◆ And finally, in 2000, Creamer et al. looked at sixty-nine subjects with knee arthritis to find out what factors were associated with functional impairment. Level of disability, pain, depression, anxiety, helplessness, self-efficacy, fatigue, quality of life, a detailed knee exam, and X rays were all evaluated. The results revealed that function in patients with knee arthritis was more determined by pain and obesity than by structural changes in the knee. Thus, they concluded that disability was unrelated to arthritic changes seen on the X-ray picture.

As all this research demonstrates, what a person's knee looks like on an X-ray picture is only weakly associated with how badly their knee hurts or how disabled they are. It may be a hard pill to swallow, but as you have just seen, many studies have arrived at identical conclusions.

Try to think of this as good news. There are currently just a few ways to change the actual structure of one's knee—one example being a joint replacement, which in all fairness can yield good results in many cases. However, the things that have been shown to be significantly associated with knee pain and disability—such as psychological variables, muscle strength, and body weight—*are* changeable. These points should be considered as practical information that knee-pain sufferers can put to good use.

> ◆ *According to much research, how a knee looks on an X-ray picture is not a sufficient explanation for the amount of pain and disability seen in patients with knee arthritis.*
>
> ◆ *The published knee literature has consistently pinpointed other factors that are linked to the level of pain and degree of disability a person has. Some of these include muscle strength, obesity, age, and psychological variables such as anxiety and depression.*

Doctors Recommend It.
The Research Says It Works. Why Not Use It?

I have some good news and some bad news for you. The bad news is that although I have brought to your attention some little-known yet well-documented psychological factors found to be closely linked to knee pain and disability, I cannot offer any specific self-help treatments for them. This is for two good reasons. The first one is that I am a physical therapist and have had little formal training in how to treat issues such as depression or anxiety. The second reason is that in my medical experience, psychological issues usually require professional assistance to be properly treated. If you feel that you have any psychological issues that might be a factor in your knee pain, please do not hesitate to seek professional help. It just may turn out to be a missing piece of the puzzle.

Time now for the good news. While I don't have any do-it-yourself treatments to specifically address the various psychological variables found to be associated with knee pain and disability, I won't leave you high and dry. I can teach you a handy mental technique that has been proven in controlled trials to quiet the mind and relieve pain. Please note that I am not including it to cure anxiety or depression, or to improve your overall psychological well-being. Rather it has been proven to help manage all sorts of acute and chronic pain conditions, and therefore it fits perfectly into this book. Sound too good to be true? Believe me, it's not. And the best part of all is that it's ridiculously easy to do!

✦ ✦ ✦ *The Relaxation Response*

Have you ever nodded out while driving a car? Maybe you left early in the morning on a long car trip or had just finished working the graveyard shift. Do you remember what happened as soon as you looked up and saw your car heading off the road? Wow, did your heart pound! Or how about the time someone snuck up behind you and scared the living daylights out of you? Can you recall the rush of adrenaline that surged through your body? These are common examples of what is popularly known as the body's *fight-or-flight response*.

Stressful situations such as these are known to trigger our built-in fight-or-flight response. Immediately, the following automatic changes take place in your body:

- ◆ your heart starts to beat faster
- ◆ your blood pressure rises
- ◆ you breathe faster
- ◆ more blood is suddenly sent to your muscles

All these changes occur in order to prepare us to either protect ourselves or run away. It's an inborn response that has been with us for thousands of years, and you can see how it serves nicely as a survival mechanism.

This brings us to what is known as the *relaxation response*. Simply put, the relaxation response is the exact opposite of the fight-or-flight response. It was popularized in the seventies by Herbert Benson, a Harvard physician, who wrote all about the topic in his best-selling book of the same name, *The Relaxation Response.*

As a young cardiologist, Dr. Benson initially became interested in the relationship between stress and high blood pressure. He eventually went on to conduct and publish much research in this area. He discovered that just as happened with the fight-or-flight response, the human body could predictably be put into an opposite state he referred to as the *relaxation response*. When a person is in this state, the following things occur:

- ◆ blood pressure drops
- ◆ breathing slows down
- ◆ heart rate decreases
- ◆ the body uses less oxygen

Dr. Benson also found that just as stress acted as a trigger for the flight-or-flight response, the relaxation response could also be reliably triggered. Ultimately, he discovered that two things were necessary to consistently induce the relaxation response. They are

- ◆ repeating a word, sound, prayer, phrase, or muscular activity and
- ◆ passively disregarding everyday thoughts that come to mind, and returning to the repetition.

Aside from being one of the most well-researched mind-body techniques around, the best thing about the relaxation response is that it is "wired" into the way our body works. Just as you do not need to believe in penicillin in order for it to work, so it is with the relaxation response.

◆ ◆ ◆ *Proven to Work on Pain*

In medicine, the word proven means that a treatment has been shown to work in a controlled trial. As discussed earlier in the book, a controlled trial is a study in which one group of people receives a treatment—say, magnets placed on the knees to relieve pain—and another group, called the control group, gets no treatment at all. At the end of the study, by comparing which group fares best, researchers can tell if the treatment (magnets, in our example) really does relieve knee pain. If the people who wore the magnets suffer less knee pain than the control group, then one could say that magnets really do help people's knee pain. On the other hand, if the people who wore magnets and the control group both get better, then we would say that magnets do not help knee pain, because whether or not a person in the study wore magnets, they got better anyway!

This example illustrates why a control group is so important in a study. Without one, researchers cannot tell if someone got better due to the new treatment they were testing or because of other factors, such as the passing of time or the placebo effect. My advice is to do what the doctors do: To determine if a treatment is really effective, find out if it has shown good results in a controlled trial.

Now that you know what I mean when I say that a treatment is proven to work, let's see what types of conditions the relaxation response has helped, when subjected to a controlled trial:

Acute and Chronic Conditions Proven to Be Helped by the Relaxation Response	
Acute pain	**Chronic pain**
after gallbladder removal	low back pain
after a hernia repair	neck pain
after a hemorrhoidectomy	shoulder pain
after an abdominal hysterectomy	arm pain
after the repair of a fractured hip	leg pain
after an episiotomy	facial pain
	headaches
	chest pain

This list was compiled from an extremely comprehensive 1996 review article on the effectiveness of the relaxation response, published in *The Journal of Cardiovascular Nursing*. As you can see, the relaxation response has been shown to be most beneficial in helping all kinds of painful conditions, both acute and chronic.

> ◆ *The relaxation response is the opposite of the body's "fight-or-flight" response mechanism.*
> ◆ *Studies have shown that the relaxation response can predictably be triggered.*
> ◆ *Many controlled trials have proven the value of the relaxation response in decreasing both acute and chronic pain.*

How to Trigger the Relaxation Response

I mentioned above that there are two essential ingredients of the relaxation response. According to Dr. Benson, they are

- ◆ repeating a word, sound, prayer, phrase, or muscular activity and

- ◆ passively disregarding everyday thoughts that come to mind and returning to the repetition.

As suggested by these two simple elements, there are many ways to evoke the relaxation response. Some interventions that have been studied and shown to trigger the relaxation response include

- ◆ meditation

- ◆ imagery

- ◆ hypnosis

- ◆ autogenic training

- ◆ progressive muscle relaxation

While these are all perfectly acceptable ways of evoking the relaxation response, I have found the following method to be by far the easiest and least complicated. Here are instructions, which have been adapted from the ones in Dr. Benson's book, *The Relaxation Response.*

- ◆ Pick a word, short phrase, or short prayer to focus on; choose something that's firmly rooted in your belief system. Examples might be "One," "Relax," or "Our Father who art in heaven."

- ◆ Sit quietly in a comfortable position, if possible, but other positions such as kneeling or standing will work as well.

- ◆ Close your eyes, if possible, but you can do it with your eyes open if you wish.

- ◆ Breathe slowly and naturally, and as you do, repeat your focus word, phrase, or prayer silently to yourself as you exhale.

- Don't worry about how well you're doing. When other thoughts come into your mind, just say, "Oh, well," and return to the repetition.

- Do this for ten to twenty minutes, once or twice daily. If necessary, gradually work up to ten or twenty minutes. Start at three to five minutes once or twice daily. Each day, see if you can add another minute to your practice.

7

Pulling It All Together: The Program That Will Work Wonders for Your Knee

The first chapter of this book explained in general terms how to treat knee pain. It put forth the theory that knee pain is the result of something failing to function properly, and that if the function is restored, the pain will go away. Then we addressed the specific knee functions that need to be restored. As you'll recall, I divided them into groups and called them "the four abilities your knee must have." They are as follows:

+ good muscular strength
+ adequate flexibility
+ working proprioception
+ enough endurance to allow the knee to perform movements over and over again

The rest of the book provided you with the tools you need in order to restore these four abilities, as well as the scientific rationale for using them. In this chapter we will pull all the information together and put it into action.

First, a Few Trade Secrets

If you were to come to me for physical therapy, you would learn that there are two supportive treatments I often use that seem to make the therapeutic exercises go smoother. They are heat and massage. I call them "supportive treatments" because they do not directly treat or correct a knee problem in and of themselves, but rather "support" the real treatment (the exercise) that follows them. An analogy I use to explain this concept is that of anesthesia. The anesthesia is a "supportive treatment" in that it doesn't directly treat or solve a problem, but it certainly makes surgery (the real treatment for the problem) go a whole lot smoother. For these reasons, whether to use heat and massage is entirely up to you. Neither is an absolutely essential part of the plan to help your knee get better.

◆ ◆ ◆ *Using Heat*

Using heat shouldn't be as big a deal as some people make it. Physical therapy clinics commonly use moist heat packs that are soaked in very hot water and afterward are wrapped in towels and placed over the knee. This method provides good heat, so if you have all the necessary supplies at your disposal, it's a suitable treatment. However, to my knowledge, there is no evidence in the literature showing that one form of heat is better than another. Therefore, use what you have available. For most people, this will probably mean using an electric heating pad or some form of microwaveable hot pack.

Here are a few tips for using heat on your knee:

◆ **Check with your doctor before using heat.** Some medical conditions prohibit the use of heat, such as conditions causing decreased sensation. In addition, if your knees have experienced sudden swelling, you shouldn't use heat on them.

- Place the heat around the whole knee, if possible.

- The purpose of using heat is to relax the knee area and its muscles before exercising; therefore, we're not really concerned that it be a specific temperature. Just make sure it feels nice and warm and is comfortable.

- I suggest applying heat for five to ten minutes. Again, the goal is simply to relax the knee, so we don't need to worry about a specific number of minutes.

◆ ◆ ◆ *Using Massage*

In my opinion, massage should follow heat, rather than vice versa. This is because muscles that have just come off heat are usually relaxed and less sore, making the massage much more effective.

More massage techniques exist than you can shake a stick at. Here again, however, scientific evidence is lacking that shows one type of massage or one particular technique as being superior for loosening muscles and increasing circulation. Therefore, I suggest a simple technique called *transverse massage*. It's so named because each muscle runs in a particular direction (just like the grain of a wood), and this massage technique has you strum transversely—that is, across the muscle tissue—as if you were playing a guitar.

Here's how it's done:

- Get into a comfortable position that will allow you to rub both the front and the back of your knee area. A sitting position on a couch, bed, or floor usually works well.

- I recommend using lotion to decrease the friction between your hand and the skin as you rub. Any ordinary hand lotion will work.

◆ With your fingers, rub back and forth across the knee muscles firmly (but comfortably) in the direction shown below, almost as if you were sawing something. Start at the knee-cap and work your way up the thigh as far as you reasonably can. Several minutes of massage should be fine.

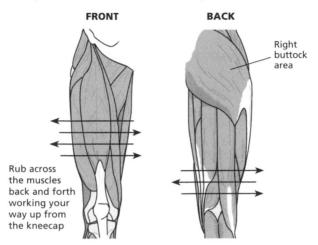

Figure 7.1 and Figure 7.2 Transverse massage of the major muscles on the front and back of the upper leg

◆ Don't be surprised if the muscles are sore in spots; a certain amount of soreness is normal during massage. And don't be surprised if the muscles feel looser after you finish.

◆ After you have massaged the front of the thigh, spend a few minutes doing the same massage on the back of the thigh.

The Master Plan

This section will help you organize all of the exercises from the preceding chapters into an easy and practical program. We'll start with an overview of a recommended schedule for you to follow:

Sunday	Monday	Tuesday	Wednesday	Thursday	Friday	Saturday
rest day	heat	heat	heat	heat	heat	rest day
	massage	massage	massage	massage	massage	
	quad-strengthening exercise		quad-strengthening exercise		quad-strengthening exercise	
	hamstring stretch	hamstring stretch	hamstring stretch	hamstring stretch	hamstring stretch	
	quad stretch	quad stretch	quad stretch	quad stretch	quad stretch	
	proprioception exercise		proprioception exercise		proprioception exercise	
	endurance exercise		endurance exercise		endurance exercise	
relaxation response	relaxation response	relaxation response	relaxation response	relaxation response	relaxation response	relaxation response

(A checklist of this plan is included in the Appendix. It follows the schedule on the previous page for six weeks. Feel free to photocopy it and keep it handy.)

Below is a closer look at each day:

◆ ◆ ◆ *Saturday and Sunday*

- *Rest* from all exercises.
- *Relaxation response (optional)*—10–20 minutes once or twice a day.

◆ ◆ ◆ *Monday, Wednesday, and Friday*

- Heat (optional)—Apply for 5–10 minutes, with knee in a comfortable position.
- *Massage (optional)*—Using lotion, start at the kneecap and rub across the muscles for several minutes, working up the thigh as far as you reasonably can. Repeat on back of leg.

QUAD-STRENGTHENING EXERCISE

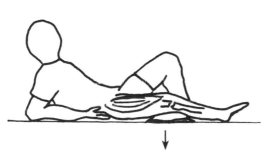

- *Quad-strengthening exercise*—Fold a pillow in half and place it under your knee. Press down as hard as you comfortably can into the pillow with your knee, and hold for 3–5 seconds. The muscle on the top of your thigh (the quadriceps) should tighten up. Work up to 30 repetitions.

HAMSTRING STRETCHES (PICK JUST ONE)

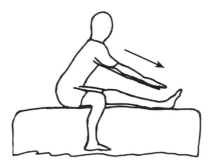

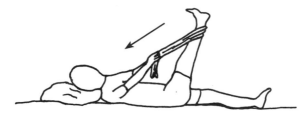

◆ *Hamstring stretch*—Get into one of the stretch positions shown above. You should feel a good but gentle stretch in the back of your leg above the knee. Hold for 30 seconds. Do once a day.

QUADRICEPS STRETCHES (PICK JUST ONE)

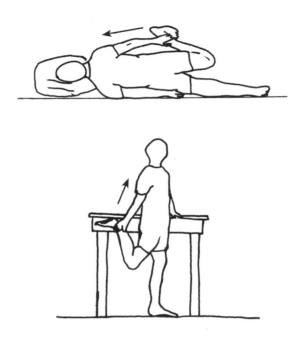

◆ *Quadriceps stretch*—Get into one of the stretch positions shown above. You should feel a good but gentle stretch in the front of your thigh. Hold for 30 seconds. Do once a day.

PROPRIOCEPTION EXERCISE

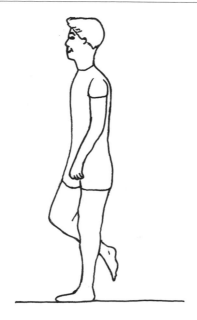

◆ *Proprioception exercise*—Stand on one leg as shown. If necessary, lightly hold on to a table, chair, or doorway for balance. Work up to standing well-balanced for a full 30 seconds, first with eyes open, then ultimately with eyes closed.

ENDURANCE EXERCISES (PICK JUST ONE)

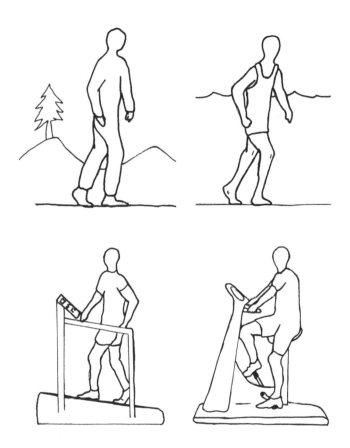

- *Endurance exercise*—Select one of the exercises shown above, and work up to doing it continuously for 20–30 minutes.

- *Relaxation response (optional)*—10–20 minutes once or twice a day.

◆ ◆ ◆ *Tuesday and Thursday*

- *Heat (optional)*—Apply for 5–10 minutes, with knee in a comfortable position.

- *Massage (optional)*—Using lotion, start at kneecap and rub across the muscles for several minutes, working up the thigh as far as you reasonably can. Repeat on back of leg.

HAMSTRING STRETCHES (PICK JUST ONE)

- *Hamstring stretch*—Get into one of the stretch positions shown on page 92. You should feel a good but gentle stretch in the back of your leg above the knee. Hold for 30 seconds. Do once a day.

QUADRICEPS STRETCHES (PICK JUST ONE)

- *Quadriceps stretch*—Get into one of the stretch positions shown on page 93. You should feel a good but gentle stretch in the front of your thigh. Hold for 30 seconds. Do once a day.

- *Relaxation response (optional)*—10–20 minutes once or twice a day.

As you can see, you do not have to exercise every day. In fact, doing all of the exercises every day will actually work against you. Rest time is every bit as important as exercising because it gives your knee time to repair and rebuild itself in order to get ready for the next workout. You may also have noticed the following:

- stretching exercises are done *five* times a week

- strengthening exercises are done *three* times a week

- endurance exercises are done *three* times a week

- proprioception exercises are done *three* times a week

As long as you follow these rules, you can shuffle things around a bit if you wish. For example, you could do your strengthening, proprioception, and endurance exercises on Tuesday, Thursday, and Saturday instead of Monday, Wednesday, and Friday, and you could stretch on any five days.

Exercise Substitutions

This book was written for the average person with knee pain who lacks access to a lot of fancy exercise equipment. The program allows you to rehabilitate your own knee with virtually no equipment. However, I realize that some readers, such as athletes, may be functioning at a high level or may indeed have access to exercise equipment and will wonder if they can substitute using some of that equipment for the exercises in this book.

Accordingly, I have included a few substitutions that will accomplish the same goals as the original exercises:

Home exercise	Substitution
Strengthening exercise: isometric quadriceps exercise using pillow	Leg extension machine (from a sitting position with bent knee, the user straightens his/her leg)
Proprioception exercise: standing on one leg	Wobble boards, balance boards
Endurance exercise: walking	Treadmills, exercise bike, elliptical machines
Flexibility exercise: quad and hamstring stretches	None

Remember, it doesn't matter whether you are a housewife or an athlete; The same principle still applies: Treat and improve your knee function to reduce your pain. The equipment or particular exercise you use is unimportant as long as it improves one of the four abilities of your knee. It doesn't matter whether you walk or use a treadmill, for example, since they both accomplish the goal of improving your knee's endurance.

Getting Started

Exactly how do you go about getting started on this plan to treat your knee pain? Here are a few suggestions:

- ◆ First, get an okay from your doctor to make sure that the exercises are safe for you to do.

- ◆ Next, take a look at the master plan (page 90), which outlines an overview for an entire week.

- ◆ Pick a day of the week on which to start.

- ◆ Once you've decided when you'll begin, review the detailed breakdown of activities for that particular day (starting on page 91) to learn what exercises to do, the suggested order in which to do them, and how to do them. If you need more detail on how to do any of the exercises, or on how to progress with them over time, review Chapters 2 through 5 for more extensive instructions.

- ◆ On the day you've chosen, jump right in and take the first step toward getting rid of that knee pain!

What to Expect

Even after I've taken a thorough medical history and physical evaluation, it can often be difficult for me to accurately predict how a person's knee will react to therapy and precisely how long it will take for him or her to start feeling better. Therefore, it is even harder for me to provide you, the reader, with this information since I am unfamiliar with your knee. However, I *can* reasonably tell you what happens to the average patient based upon my clinical experience and the results of many clinical studies that have used similar exercise routines. This section describes some typical scenarios and offers further information. Don't be disappointed if your experience isn't identical to what I present here; every patient is different.

You shouldn't have much difficulty doing the exercises. I have taken great care to use exercises that have been shown in clinical studies not only to be effective, but also to be well tolerated by most knee-pain patients, even those with arthritic changes in their knees. If a patient does run into problems (i.e., it hurts too much to do an exercise), most of the time it is with one of the stretches. My advice is that you be patient and keep working with the stretches (or any of the other exercises) unless you either experience a big increase in pain levels or notice sudden swelling. A little increase in discomfort and soreness is to be expected until your knee adjusts to the new range of motion and activities. At the same time, remember that it's your knee and you know it better than anybody else. Most people can distinguish discomfort caused by doing an exercise from pain that is telling them something serious is going on. Always see your doctor if in doubt.

If I dare throw out an estimate, about 25 percent of people start to notice decreased knee pain for various reasons within the first week of starting this program. The other 75 percent get better as the function of their knee improves. For example, as the knee gets stronger and more flexible, the pain gradually decreases. But this takes time, usually a period of weeks. For those of you who like numbers, six weeks is usually enough time for me to be able to clinically measure good gains in knee strength, flexibility, and the other functions. If you have followed this program by the book for three months and have noticed absolutely no change in either pain frequency or intensity, then this program is not the solution to your knee pain.

How long should you continue with the exercises? I recommend doing the full program for at least six to eight weeks. Studies show that this is how long it takes to make good, measurable gains in knee function. If your knee feels great after six to eight weeks, try doing the strengthening, stretching, proprioception, and endurance exercises one time a week for maintenance and see how that goes. If you have good pain relief by six to eight weeks but you're not quite where you want to be, continue with the program until either you reach your goal or no further progress is being made. And, as mentioned earlier, if you have not seen a lick of progress in either pain frequency or intensity after doing the program by the book for three months, then it is not the solution to your knee pain.

In Closing

Beside my desk at the hospital where I work are literally hundreds of medical articles from peer-reviewed journals that I have read over the years and that I have organized by subject in black binders. This is the foundation of my physical-therapy practice and also the source from which I have pulled all the information I included for you in this book. I hope I have succeeded in giving you some useful "tools" to help you with your knee pain. All that is left now is for you to jump right in and give that knee of yours a "tune-up." While this may be the end of the book, I prefer that you think of it as just the beginning for you and your knee. Good luck. I have enjoyed sharing the information in this book with you.

Appendix

Suggested Weekly Program: A Checklist

To help you incorporate the program into your daily schedule, you may wish to use the handy checklist pages that follow.

◆ ◆ ◆ *Week 1*

Sunday	Monday	Tuesday	Wednesday	Thursday	Friday	Saturday
☐ rest day	☐ heat (optional)	☐ heat (optional)	☐ heat (optional)	☐ heat (optional)	☐ heat (optional)	☐ rest day
☐ relaxation response (optional)	☐ massage (optional)	☐ massage (optional)	☐ massage (optional)	☐ massage (optional)	☐ massage (optional)	☐ relaxation response (optional)
	☐ quad-strengthening exercise	☐ hamstring stretch	☐ quad-strengthening exercise	☐ hamstring stretch	☐ quad-strengthening exercise	
	☐ hamstring stretch	☐ quad stretch	☐ hamstring stretch	☐ quad stretch	☐ hamstring stretch	
	☐ quad stretch	☐ relaxation response (optional)	☐ quad stretch	☐ relaxation response (optional)	☐ quad stretch	
	☐ proprioception exercise		☐ proprioception exercise		☐ proprioception exercise	
	☐ endurance exercise		☐ endurance exercise		☐ endurance exercise	
	☐ relaxation response (optional)		☐ relaxation response (optional)		☐ relaxation response (optional)	

◆ ◆ ◆ *Week 2*

Sunday	Monday	Tuesday	Wednesday	Thursday	Friday	Saturday
☐ rest day	☐ heat (optional)	☐ heat (optional)	☐ heat (optional)	☐ heat (optional)	☐ heat (optional)	☐ rest day
☐ relaxation response (optional)	☐ massage (optional)	☐ massage (optional)	☐ massage (optional)	☐ massage (optional)	☐ massage (optional)	☐ relaxation response (optional)
	☐ quad-strengthening exercise	☐ hamstring stretch	☐ quad-strengthening exercise	☐ hamstring stretch	☐ quad-strengthening exercise	
	☐ hamstring stretch	☐ quad stretch	☐ hamstring stretch	☐ quad stretch	☐ hamstring stretch	
	☐ quad stretch	☐ relaxation response (optional)	☐ quad stretch	☐ relaxation response (optional)	☐ quad stretch	
	☐ proprioception exercise		☐ proprioception exercise		☐ proprioception exercise	
	☐ endurance exercise		☐ endurance exercise		☐ endurance exercise	
	☐ relaxation response (optional)		☐ relaxation response (optional)		☐ relaxation response (optional)	

◆ ◆ ◆ *Week 3*

Sunday	Monday	Tuesday	Wednesday	Thursday	Friday	Saturday
☐ rest day	☐ heat (optional)	☐ heat (optional)	☐ heat (optional)	☐ heat (optional)	☐ heat (optional)	☐ rest day
☐ relaxation response (optional)	☐ massage (optional)	☐ massage (optional)	☐ massage (optional)	☐ massage (optional)	☐ massage (optional)	☐ relaxation response (optional)
	☐ quad-strength-ening exercise	☐ hamstring stretch	☐ quad-strength-ening exercise	☐ hamstring stretch	☐ quad-strength-ening exercise	
	☐ hamstring stretch	☐ quad stretch	☐ hamstring stretch	☐ quad stretch	☐ hamstring stretch	
	☐ quad stretch	☐ relaxation response (optional)	☐ quad stretch	☐ relaxation response (optional)	☐ quad stretch	
	☐ proprioception exercise		☐ proprioception exercise		☐ proprioception exercise	
	☐ endurance exercise		☐ endurance exercise		☐ endurance exercise	
	☐ relaxation response (optional)		☐ relaxation response (optional)		☐ relaxation response (optional)	

◆ ◆ ◆ *Week 4*

Sunday	Monday	Tuesday	Wednesday	Thursday	Friday	Saturday
☐ rest day	☐ heat (optional)	☐ heat (optional)	☐ heat (optional)	☐ heat (optional)	☐ heat (optional)	☐ rest day
☐ relaxation response (optional)	☐ massage (optional)	☐ massage (optional)	☐ massage (optional)	☐ massage (optional)	☐ massage (optional)	☐ relaxation response (optional)
	☐ quad-strengthening exercise	☐ hamstring stretch	☐ quad-strengthening exercise	☐ hamstring stretch	☐ quad-strengthening exercise	
	☐ hamstring stretch	☐ quad stretch	☐ hamstring stretch	☐ quad stretch	☐ hamstring stretch	
	☐ quad stretch	☐ relaxation response (optional)	☐ quad stretch	☐ relaxation response (optional)	☐ quad stretch	
	☐ proprioception exercise		☐ proprioception exercise		☐ proprioception exercise	
	☐ endurance exercise		☐ endurance exercise		☐ endurance exercise	
	☐ relaxation response (optional)		☐ relaxation response (optional)		☐ relaxation response (optional)	

◆ ◆ *Week 5*

Sunday	Monday	Tuesday	Wednesday	Thursday	Friday	Saturday
□ rest day	□ heat (optional)	□ heat (optional)	□ heat (optional)	□ heat (optional)	□ heat (optional)	□ rest day
□ relaxation response (optional)	□ massage (optional)	□ massage (optional)	□ massage (optional)	□ massage (optional)	□ massage (optional)	□ relaxation response (optional)
	□ quad-strengthening exercise	□ hamstring stretch	□ quad-strengthening exercise	□ hamstring stretch	□ quad-strengthening exercise	
	□ hamstring stretch	□ quad stretch	□ hamstring stretch	□ quad stretch	□ hamstring stretch	
	□ quad stretch	□ relaxation response (optional)	□ quad stretch	□ relaxation response (optional)	□ quad stretch	
	□ proprioception exercise		□ proprioception exercise		□ proprioception exercise	
	□ endurance exercise		□ endurance exercise		□ endurance exercise	
	□ relaxation response (optional)		□ relaxation response (optional)		□ relaxation response (optional)	

◆ ◆ ◆ *Week 6*

Sunday	Monday	Tuesday	Wednesday	Thursday	Friday	Saturday
☐ rest day	☐ heat (optional)	☐ heat (optional)	☐ heat (optional)	☐ heat (optional)	☐ heat (optional)	☐ rest day
☐ relaxation response (optional)	☐ massage (optional)	☐ massage (optional)	☐ massage (optional)	☐ massage (optional)	☐ massage (optional)	☐ relaxation response (optional)
	☐ quad-strengthening exercise	☐ hamstring stretch	☐ quad-strengthening exercise	☐ hamstring stretch	☐ quad-strengthening exercise	
	☐ hamstring stretch	☐ quad stretch	☐ hamstring stretch	☐ quad stretch	☐ hamstring stretch	
	☐ quad stretch	☐ relaxation response (optional)	☐ quad stretch	☐ relaxation response (optional)	☐ quad stretch	
	☐ proprioception exercise		☐ proprioception exercise		☐ proprioception exercise	
	☐ endurance exercise		☐ endurance exercise		☐ endurance exercise	
	☐ relaxation response (optional)		☐ relaxation response (optional)		☐ relaxation response (optional)	

References

Introduction

Thomas, K. S., et al. "Home Based Exercise Programme for Knee Pain and Knee Osteoarthritis: Randomized Controlled Trial." *British Medical Journal* 325:752–55, 2002.

Topp, Robert, et al. "The Effect of Dynamic Versus Isometric Resistance Training on Pain and Functioning among Adults with Osteoarthritis of the Knee." *Archives of Physical Medicine and Rehabilitation* 83:1187–95, 2002.

Chapter 2

Carolan, B., and Cafarelli, E. "Adaptations in Coactivation after Isometric Resistance Training." *Journal of Applied Physiology* 73(3):911–17, 1992.

Fahrer, H., et al. "Knee Effusion and Reflex Inhibition of the Quadriceps: A Bar to Effective Retraining." *Journal of Bone and Joint Surgery [Br]* 70-B: 635–38, 1988.

Garfinkel, S., and Carafelli, E. "Relative Changes in Maximal Force, EMG, and Muscle Cross-Sectional Area after Isometric Training." *Medicine and Science in Sports and Exercise* 24(11):1220–27, 1992.

Gerber, C., et al. "The Lower-Extremity Musculature in Chronic Symptomatic Instability of the Anterior Cruciate Ligament." *Journal of Bone and Joint Surgery* 67-A:1034–43, 1985.

Hassan, B. S., et al. "Static Postural Sway, Proprioception, and Maximal Voluntary Quadriceps Contraction in Patients with Knee Osteoarthritis and Normal Control Subjects." *Annals of the Rheumatic Diseases* 60:612–18, 2001.

Hurley, M. V., and Newham D. J. "The Influence of Arthrogenous Muscle Inhibition on Quadriceps Rehabilitation of Patients with Early, Unilateral Osteoarthritic Knees." *British Journal of Rheumatology* 32:127–31, 1993.

Lopresti, C., et al. "Degree of Quadriceps Atrophy at One Year Post Anterior Cruciate Repair." *Medicine and Science in Sports and Exercise* 16:204, 1984.

Manal, Tara J., and Snyder-Mackler, L. "Failure of Voluntary Activation of the Quadriceps Femoris Muscle after Patellar Contusion." *Journal of Orthopedic and Sports Physical Therapy* 30(11):654–63, 2000.

Slemenda, C., et al. "Quadriceps Weakness and Osteoarthritis of the Knee." *Annals of Internal Medicine* 127:97–104, 1997.

Slemenda, C., et al. "Reduced Quadriceps Strength Relative to Body Weight: A Risk Factor for Knee Osteoarthritis in Women?" *Arthritis and Rheumatism* 41(11):1951–59, 1998.

Spencer, Jennifer D., et al. "Knee Joint Effusion and Quadriceps Reflex Inhibition in Man." *Archives of Physical Medicine and Rehabilitation* 65:171–77, 1984.

Stener, B., and Petersen, I. "Electromyographic Investigation of Reflex Effects upon Stretching the Partially Ruptured Medial Collateral Ligament of the Knee Joint." *Acta Chirurgica Scandinavica* 124:396–415, 1962.

Stener, Bertil. "Reflex Inhibition of the Quadriceps Elicited from a Subperiosteal Tumour of the Femur." *Acta Orthopaedica Scandinavica* 40:86–91, 1969.

Young, A., et al. "Measurement of Quadriceps Muscle Wasting by Ultrasonography." *Rheumatology and Rehabilitation* 19(3):141–48, 1980.

Chapter 3

American Academy of Orthopedic Surgeons. *Joint Motion: Method of Measuring and Recording.* Chicago: AAOS, 1965.

Bandy, W. D., Irion, J. M. "The Effect of Time on Static Stretch on the Flexibility of the Hamstring Muscles." *Physical Therapy* 74:845–52, 1994.

Bandy, W. D., et al. "The Effect of Time and Frequency of Static Stretching on Flexibility of the Hamstring Muscles." *Physical Therapy* 77:1090–1096, 1997.

Clark, W. A. "A System of Joint Measurement." *J Orthop Surg* 2:687, 1920.

Daniels, L., and Worthingham, C. *Muscle Testing: Techniques of Manual Examination*, 3d ed. Philadelphia, WB Saunders: 1972.

Escalante, A., et al. "Walking Velocity in Aged Persons: Its Association with Lower Extremity Joint Range of Motion." *Arthritis Care and Research* 45: 287–94, 2001.

Helfet, A. J. "Mechanism of Derangements of the Medial Semilunar Cartilage and Their Management." *Journal of Bone and Joint Surgery (Br.)* 41-B(2):319–36, 1959.

Journal of the American Medical Association: A Guide to the Evaluation of Permanent Impairment of the Extremities and Back (special ed.) 1, 1958.

Kapandji, I. A. *Physiology of the Joints*, vols. 1 and 2, 2d ed. London: Churchill Livingstone, 1970.

Kendall, F. P., and McCreary, E. K. *Muscles: Testing and Function*, 3d ed. Baltimore: Williams and Wilkins, 1983.

Rowe, P. J., et al. "Knee Joint Kinematics in Gait and Other Functional Activities Measured Using Flexible Electrogoniometry: How Much Knee Motion Is Sufficient for Normal Daily Life?" *Gait and Posture* 12:143–55, 2000.

Chapter 4

Baker, V., et al. "Abnormal Knee Joint Position Sense in Individuals with Patellofemoral Pain Syndrome." *Journal of Orthopedic Research* 20(2):208–14, 2002.

Caraffa, A., et al. "Prevention of Anterior Cruciate Ligament Injuries in Soccer: A Prospective Controlled Study of Proprioceptive Training." *Knee Surgery, Sports Traumatology, Arthroscopy* 4(1):19–21, 1996.

Fischer-Rasmussen, T., and Jensen, P. E. "Proprioceptive Sensitivity and Performance in Anterior Cruciate Ligament–Deficient Knee Joints." *Scandanavian Journal of Medicine and Science in Sports* 10(2):85–89, 2000.

Hassan, B. S., et al. "Static Postural Sway, Proprioception, and Maximal Voluntary Quadriceps Contraction in Patients with Knee Osteoarthritis and Normal Control Subjects." *Annals of the Rheumatic Diseases* 60(6):612–18, 2001.

Jerosch, J., and Prymka, M. "Knee Joint Proprioception in Patients with Posttraumatic Recurrent Patella Dislocation." *Knee Surgery, Sports Traumatology, Arthroscopy* 4(1):14–18, 1996.

Jerosch, J., and Prymka, M. "Proprioceptive Deficits of the Knee Joint after Rupture of the Medial Meniscus." *Unfallchirurg* 100(6):444–48, 1997.

Petrella, R. J., et al. "Effect of Age and Activity on Knee Joint Proprioception." *American Journal of Physical Medicine and Rehabilitation* 76(3):235–41, 1997.

Chapter 5

www.guinnessworldrecords.com

Messier, S. P., et al. "Etiologic Factors Associated with Patellofemoral Pain in Runners." *Medicine and Science in Sports and Exercise* 23(9):1008–15, 1991.

Schwendner, K. I., et al. "Differences in Muscle Endurance and Recovery Between Fallers and Nonfallers, and Between Young and Older Women. *Journals of Gerontology Series A-Biological Sciences and Medical Sciences* 52(3):M155–60, 1997.

Chapter 6

Bagge, E., et al. "Osteoarthritis in the Elderly: Clinical and Radiological Findings in 79 and 85 Year Olds." *Annals of the Rheumatic Diseases* 50:535–39, 1991.

Benson, H. *The Relaxation Response*. New York: Harper Torch, 1975.

Boden, S., et al. "A Prospective and Blinded Investigation of Magnetic Resonance Imaging of the Knee: Abnormal Findings in Asymptomatic Subjects." *Clinical Orthopedics and Related Research* 282:177–85, 1992.

Brunner, Michael C., et al. "MRI of the Athletic Knee: Findings in Asymptomatic Professional Basketball and Collegiate Football Players." *Investigative Radiology* 24:72–75, 1989.

Creamer, P., et al. "Factors Associated with Functional Impairment in Symptomatic Knee Osteoarthritis." *Rheumatology* 39:490–96, 2000.

Felson, David T., et al. "The Prevalence of Knee Osteoarthritis in the Elderly: The Framingham Osteoarthritis Study." *Arthritis and Rheumatism* 30(8):914–18, 1987.

Kornick, Jeffrey, et al. "Meniscal Abnormalities in the Asymptomatic Population at MR Imaging." *Radiology* 177:463–65, 1990.

Lawrence, J. S., et al. "Osteo-arthrosis: Prevalence in the Population and Relationship Between Symptoms and X-Ray Changes." *Annals of the Rheumatic Diseases* 25:1–24, 1966.

Mandle, Carol Lynn, et al. "The Efficacy of Relaxation Response Interventions with Adult Patients: A Review of the Literature." *Journal of Cardiovascular Nursing* 10(3):4–26, 1996.

Massardo, L., et al. "Osteoarthritis of the Knee Joint: An Eight-Year Prospective Study." *Annals of the Rheumatic Diseases* 48:893–97, 1989.

McAlindon, T. E., et al. "Determinants of Disability in Osteoarthritis of the Knee." *Annals of the Rheumatic Diseases* 52:258–62, 1993.

Reginster, J. Y., et al. "Joint Space Narrowing Is Poorly Correlated with Symptoms Worsening in Knee Osteoarthritis: Results from the Prospective Follow-Up of 106, Placebo-Treated Patients for Three Years." Highlights from the 2002 Annual European Congress of Rheumatology. Available at: http://www.hopkins-arthritis.som.jhmi.edu/edu/eular2002/oa-clinical-rad.html. Accessed February 17, 2003.

Salaffi, Fausto, et al. "Analysis of Disability in Knee Osteoarthritis: Relationship with Age and Psychological Variables but Not with Radiographic Score." *Journal of Rheumatology* 18:1581–86, 1991.

Shellock, Frank G., et al. "Do Asymptomatic Marathon Runners Have an Increased Prevalence of Meniscal Abnormalities? An MR Study of the Knee in 23 Volunteers." *American Journal of Roentgenology* 157:1239–41, 1991.

Summers, Mary N., et al. "Radiographic Assessment and Psychologic Variables as Predictors of Pain and Functional Impairment in Osteoarthritis of the Knee or Hip." *Arthritis and Rheumatism* 31(2):204–9, 1988.

Van Baar, Margriet E., et al. "Pain and Disability in Patients with Osteoarthritis of Hip or Knee: The Relationship with Articular, Kinesiological, and Psychological Characteristics." *Journal of Rheumatology* 25:125–33, 1998.

Resources

American Academy of Orthopaedic Surgeons
Public service telephone number: (800) 824-BONES (2663)
http://orthoinfo.aaos.org

The site provides fact sheets on many orthopedic conditions and treatments including specific knee problems. Reviewed by doctors to ensure medical accuracy.

National Library of Medicine ◆ www.nlm.nih.gov

This site is brought to you by the National Library of Medicine, which also happens to be the world's largest medical library! Here you can get access to some of the huge medical databases that I regularly use to search for scientific articles.

Medline Plus Health Information ◆ www.medlineplus.gov

This site contains information on numerous health topics, as well as drug information, a medical encyclopedia/dictionary, current health news, and a directory to find doctors, dentists, and hospitals.

American Physical Therapy Association ◆ www.apta.org

This site contains an online directory of Certified Clinical Specialists in various areas of physical therapy (in this case, orthopedics for a knee specialist) so you can locate the one nearest you.

ClinicalTrials.gov ◆ www.clinicaltrials.gov

A service of the National Institutes of Health, this site gives information on the latest clinical trials being conducted for many health conditions. Here you can type in "knee pain" and see the current research that is being conducted as well as how you can participate in some these studies.

Index

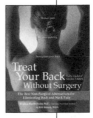
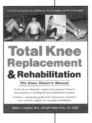
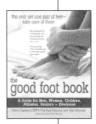

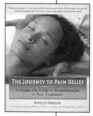
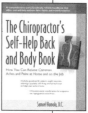
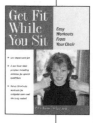